Life,
Longevity,
and The Kiso Diet™

Dr. Craig Zion Cain

Published by Kiso Life Systems

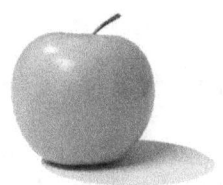

It's not a diet. It's a Lifestyle.

Life, Longevity and The Kiso Diet™
Craig Zion Cain, D.C.
Published by Kiso Life Systems
www.KisoDiet.com
© 2011

ISBN 978-1461164494

Printed in the United States of America

Editing, layout and cover design by Leslie Sears
Les is More Printing & Graphics, Hilo, Hawaii

Dedication

For my wife, Eika,

who prepared a kiso diet daily in our home,

long before **The Kiso Diet™** was ever written...

Foreword by Gilad

*Most people know me through my daily fitness show **Bodies In Motion™** and my **Total Body Sculpt** workouts. The fact is, I have been into athletics for as long as I can remember. I competed in track and field in the Decathlon on an international level in my late teens and early twenties.*

Over the years, pursuing and advocating a healthy and fit lifestyle to my viewers and participants, I've been blessed with the opportunity to meet and work with other passionate health professionals. I met Dr. Cain on the island of Hawaii, and was taken by his knowledge and desire to help people through his message of healthy eating and disease-preventing nutritional diets. We ended up working together during my first public fitness camp with great success. Our participants loved his informative and easy to understand principals. Many of them took the information home with them and applied it to their daily lives.

As a "health nut" myself, Dr. Cain's message resonates with me loud and clear. Anyone can dramatically improve his or her life by applying simple and easy to follow dietary principals. From my perspective, there is no true fitness without a healthy diet at its core.

Preface

Kiso in Japanese means **"foundation of internal energy."** I call the healing process I created the **Kiso Method™.**

Human beings are energy beings. The more balanced energy we store and possess, the better we feel. Kiso Method™ is a form of healing practiced by chiropractors, massage therapists, and cranio-sacral therapists to remove energy blocks and restore balance.[1]

Kiso Method™ gently rids the body of nerve impingements, allowing the cranial-sacral system to function normally. Getting rid of energy blockers in the spine allows your immune system to have more energy and do its job better. The alignment of the cranial-sacral system makes the two parts of our nervous systems, the *para-sympathetic* and the *sympathetic* nervous systems, act in conjunction. We need both to function normally; not one operating in sympathetic

---

[1] The principals of the Kiso Method™ are put into a book for the lay-person called **Secrets of Healing Back Pain.** The Kiso Method™ with manuals 1 & 2 are available in our book called **Kiso Method, Structural Alignment**. You can find them on Amazon.com, or on our website, www.kisomethod.com.

override, causing adrenal burnout, anxiety, and possible panic attacks. The Kiso Method™ healing process addresses these issues and more, dramatically helping even people who suffer from chronic pain.

For years in my clinics practicing the Kiso Method™, I brought people into balance, and sent them off to live their normal lives. But I felt there should be more... After a person had been cleared and balanced, it just did not make sense to have them return to their daily lives without changing the patterns that had created their health issues. I wanted them to do the rest... I wanted them to **eat right**!

That's why I became so interested in sharing what I knew about diet...or ways of eating. So I taught nutrition at the **Traditional Chinese Medical College of Hawaii**, an accredited Oriental Medicine Master's degree program, I sifted through countless diets and practices of eating to come up with what I thought was the best overall diet plan. I wrote *Life, Longevity, and the Kiso Diet*™ to share my findings.

Introduction

The viscosity, or thickness, of your blood is a major determining factor in your overall health. The Kiso Diet™ looks at eating habits as one of the major determining factors of **blood viscosity**. Diets high in saturated fats and cholesterol result in blood that is sticky and thick, making it difficult for the blood to oxygenate all areas of the body. This creates hypoxia (lack of oxygen), especially in areas of the body that require heavy oxygenation.

High blood viscosity causes a well-known disease called atherosclerosis. Maybe you've heard of this? Of course you have, atherosclerosis is always talked about in the news as a primary factor in heart disease. But did you know that the process of atherosclerosis doesn't just target the heart? It manifests throughout the body!

The lack of nutrients and oxygen causes degeneration to your joints, brain, and many other parts of your body that previously have not been associated with atherosclerosis! So it's not just our heart that's affected; our brain, organs and joints also suffer when the blood has high viscosity. A little known fact is the connection between blood viscosity, atherosclerosis, and joint pain and subsequent degeneration. From a chiropractic standpoint, that's huge. From an aging standpoint it's even bigger. We will examine this connection in depth.

Another area of focus is the connection between **milk and cancer**. **The more milk you drink, the higher your chances of getting cancer.** Not only does drinking milk make your **blood thicker** because of the saturated fats it contains, there's an added culprit: casein protein. 80% of milk's protein is casein. Casein protein circulating in the body acts like a cancer fertilizer, promoting cancer in both men and women. Not only is milk bad from a cancer standpoint, it's also a significant factor in **autoimmune diseases.** Milk has been linked to rheumatoid arthritis, multiple sclerosis, as well as thyroid diseases.

The Kiso Diet™ as a "Culture"

The Kiso Diet™ approaches eating in a cultural sense. If you have been raised with healthy cultural eating practices, you needn't "think" about every aspect of the food you eat everyday. **You don't count calories** or have a hard and fast set of "must eats" at every meal. If you look at these cultural practices you see that people are relaxed about the way they eat. They are used to eating certain foods and combining certain foods together. They just... do it!

For example, in China, they traditionally eat a low amount of meat and use milk sparingly or not at all. Of course, in olden times and in rural China, they did not eat lots of meat or drink milk because of the lack of availability. In current day China, access to foods has changed but the cultural diet has not. They don't think about it day-to-day, they just make choices that **follow their "culture" of how and what to eat**. Their geographic area helped mold their particular cultural eating habits.

Why don't Americans have a cultural diet? **Because ALL foods and beverages abound in every store in America**. There are no guidelines dictated by availability or lifestyle, at least not healthy ones. We're left to make our own choices, often dictated by cravings, advertising, and misinformation.

In the Kiso Diet™, I **EDUCATE** you on what to eat, what not to eat, and what to choose in your diet on a day-to-day basis. I educate you based on **scientific fact, research, and experimentation resulting in new compelling evidence for a healthy diet**. This new evidence and experimentation was done by **real scientists**, pursuing real results - not scientists persuaded by corporate interests to reach a specific outcome (ie: "milk does a body good"). The evidence speaks for itself.

Life, Longevity, and the Kiso Diet™ teaches you **what to eat, what to avoid,** and how you can **modify** the Kiso Diet™ to suit your tastes and lifestyle. So here goes, we're on to a new culture in America, a new beginning called **The Kiso Diet**™!

Table of Contents

Chapter 1

Life and Longevity

Life

I have used the word "**Life**" in my book title. By this I mean living life to its fullest potential by keeping your energy levels high. If your energy level is high, your *immune system* functions at its best.

Have you noticed that when you become stressed about something personal, in a few days time you might develop a skin rash, or see pimples popping up on your body? You might get a sore throat or an ear infection, joint pains, or headaches. *This is due to your immune system not functioning properly.* Your immune system will start to let bacteria, viruses, and fungus or yeasts move in. Instead of the immune system stopping these various potential problems, it lets these guys pass through *your firewall.* Yes, it's like your computer. If your virus protection on your computer is weak, it will let things pass into your system that will immediately disrupt your software program. If these problems are allowed to persist, you will find your hard drive has been infected and now it needs to be replaced! Don't let this happen to your body! Keep your body's hardware working well by keeping your immune system functioning properly. That means eating right, getting enough sleep (but not too much!), and keeping stress away!

Longevity

Longevity does not mean living until 120 (which is possible) while being sick half the time, it means living a *long healthy life vibrantly!*

One thing that study and research have shown is that if you have a healthy diet, you will live a longer life without ill health. Living to 85 but being unable to go out in the yard, unable to drive, and unable to muster the energy to walk around the block is sad. People who *eat well* tend to die more suddenly after a long life, and up until their death they have plenty of energy. They stayed off medications because they didn't need them. They were not only able to walk around the block, but many climbed mountains, attended yoga classes, practiced tai chi, and walked their dogs to death, having tons of energy! *Now which life do you want?* No energy, weak immune system, in and out of hospitals until you finally, slowly, die miserably? (Not to mention; this is hard on your loved ones.) Or, would you rather live a long life without medications, full of energy and possibility? I do believe you will pick the high energy choice.

There's a story about a man in Japan who started climbing mountains after his 70th birthday. Before age 70 he had never climbed a mountain in his life, but he became an expert mountain climber and continued to climb until well after the age of 90. Yes, he finally died, as we all will, but he lived life to its fullest and achieved a dream in the last decades of his life. Contrast this with having diabetes at the age of 7 or having heart disease at the age of 30, or multiple sclerosis and arthritis in your twenties. AAAAH, no thanks. But even if you have these diseases now, you can begin to turn things around by changing your diet. Many healing centers around the world claim to "cure" type-two diabetes in as little as 7 days! Also, there is strong evidence that multiple sclerosis and arthritis are caused by your bodies reaction to milk proteins in your blood stream. Wow!

Besides eating a healthy diet, are there other things one can do to increase longevity? Keep your stress at a minimum throughout your life. Don't sweat the small stuff. Learn how to release negative emotion and engage in a life-long practice like meditation, tai chi, yoga, or qui gong that not only keeps your mind sharp but also helps keep your body in top shape.

Did you know that exercise and muscle resistance training decrease your chances of getting cancer? *Yes, by more than 50%!* How does exercise decrease cancer risk? Because it increases the body's need for protein. Why would increasing the body's need for protein decrease cancer risk? *Good question…* Because most cancers are fertilized by having excess proteins in the body. Having an excess of protein, specifically ANIMAL protein, circulating in the body has been shown to increase the acidity of the body, promoting tumors and cancer. Eliminating excess protein, either by consuming less or by increasing the amount the body uses, is an important key to living longer.

Let's put this all together now, and begin our study of *The Kiso Diet™.*

Chapter 2

Phases of the Kiso Diet™

The Kiso Diet™ has three phases.

Phase One is the **Vegan** diet. Vegans are vegetarians who do not eat any foods derived from animal sources, including eggs, dairy or meat. Most vegans also do not use products that contain animal derivatives, including leather, fur, and wool.

On the Kiso Diet™, we use eating vegan for *cleansing and healing*. A vegan diet, which is great for healing an ailment, has been shown to actually become unhealthy if a person stays on the diet for a long period of time, say for one year or more. Why? Many find a vegan diet is too restrictive to live on comfortably, and some folks just don't eat the right combinations of foods to stay properly nourished.

But vegan diets are *cleansing and healing*, especially when used to heal a specific ailment or disease like *diabetes* or *cancer*. **The Kiso Diet™** uses it to cleanse the body. Instead of starving to death or drinking water with lemons for two weeks, just go on a vegan diet and continue to juice, that's cleansing enough. You can also substitute a vegan diet with a "raw food diet," which is also vegan, by the way. It's even harder to follow than a traditional vegan diet, but incredibly cleansing!

Everyone beginning the Kiso Diet™ is encouraged to start their first week on a vegan diet. Reading labels on food products is a must for vegans, so you will become aware of how milk and dairy products are hidden in various food products. It also acts to change your tongue. If you've been eating the SAD diet (standard American diet), you're used to a bad diet full of rich, fat, overly sweet foods. Eating cleanly sometimes takes a while to adjust to, especially for your taste buds. But once you become acclimated to it, you will prefer it!

Phase Two of the Kiso Diet™ is a **Vegetarian** diet. It's a *lacto-ovo vegetarian* diet to be exact, meaning you eat vegetarian (no meat, fish or poultry) with the addition of eggs and some dairy products. Again, we **generally avoid milk and cheese** for health reasons, but you can still eat some, just not a ton of it. This limits the risks associated with casein protein, and also cuts down on your consumption of the calories and saturated fats found in milk and cheese. You can flavor your coffee or tea with milk, but don't "drink" milk. If you like a bit of parmesan cheese on your pasta, you can have it. It's a more tasty, varied diet than eating vegan or raw foods, and it makes going out to eat a lot easier.

If you're not committed to a vegan lifestyle, after one week of eating vegan on the Kiso Diet™, you are encouraged to eat as a lacto-ovo vegetarian for one week. Again, it acclimates your taste buds and it gets you used to shopping and eating on a vegetarian diet before moving on to a broader diet, if you are so inclined.

Phase Three of the Kiso Diet™ is the **Flexitarian** diet. I use the term "Flexitarian" to describe a flexible diet, based on the healthy practices of a vegetarian lifestyle, without the rigidity. You can enjoy the added variety, nutrition, and taste of an omnivore's diet. Flexitarian diet means you can even eat meat if you want, but how often you can eat meat depends on your need for protein. At this point in the Kiso Diet™ program, you have already eaten as a vegan and as a vegetarian, so when you incorporate meat into your diet now, you will comfortably do so sparingly.

How much need for protein does a body have? Good question! I'm glad you asked! **About 10 to 12% of your daily intake of total calories should be in the form of protein**. Most Americans eat more than 20% of their total caloric intake of food in the form of protein.

What increases your body's need for protein? **Exercise! That's why Exercise is a part of the Kiso Diet™.** How much exercise is recommended? The minimum amount of exercise is **30 minutes every day, or one hour 3 times a week.** This exercise can be in the form of walking, jogging, aerobics or what ever you like doing. Just get your heart rate up to 60% of your maximum. This means while exercising you can still talk, but any more effort and you could not talk because you would be out of breath.

If you follow this *minimum exercise requirement,* you can eat meat (fish or foul is recommended over other meats) **three times a week.** Now here's the kicker, remember, your need for protein goes up with exercise. If you exercise another 15 to 20 minutes or more of *intense exercise,* like weight lifting, aerobics, running, or something that gets your heart rate up to over 60 or 70% of your maximum heart rate, you can have another "meat" on that day you exercised. Pushing it a bit more from 60% to 70% requires you work your muscles more. This causes them to break down a bit, requiring more protein for repair. But even if you exercise everyday, you can still only eat meat **once a day,** and leave one day a week totally **vegetarian or vegan.**   **Eating no more than one "meat" a day is a key part of the Kiso Diet™.**

Following this diet ensures that you will not get too much protein causing ill health and high cholesterol which not only leads to heart disease but also cancer!   Following this diet *makes* you want to work out. You can *earn* your right to eat meat proteins. **FOLLOWING THIS DIET MAKES YOU FEEL FANTASTIC!**

Chapter 3

Disease and the Standard American Diet (SAD)

The diet/health connection

More than 910,000 Americans die of heart disease annually, according to the American Heart Association. And more than 70 million Americans live every day with some form of heart disease, which can include high blood pressure, cardiovascular disease, stroke, angina (chest pain), heart attack and congenital heart defects. That's almost one third of the people in America, folks, and that's just the recorded and documented cases!

Heart attacks are the leading cause of death and illness in the United States. At the root of the cause for heart attacks is a disease called **"atherosclerosis,"** which is the accumulation of **plaque** (cholesterol, fatty deposits, and other substances) on the inner lining of artery walls. This buildup narrows arteries until they become so clogged, blood cannot flow through. This can result in death or damage to part of the heart muscle, basically causing a heart attack.

Cancer is the second leading cause of death. Colorectal and breast cancer head the list. As we will see, milk, milk protein and animal proteins are the biggest reasons for cancer.

Stroke, the third leading cause of death in America, could accurately be called a "brain attack." It happens the same exact way a heat attack and heart disease happens, by the accumulation of plaque on the lining of blood vessels and arteries, atherosclerosis. But with strokes, the atherosclerosis occurs in the arteries and vessels of the brain.

There are two main types of stroke. One, **ischemic stroke**, is caused by blockage of a blood vessel; the other, **hemorrhagic stroke**, is caused by bleeding. Bleeding strokes have a much higher death rate than strokes caused by clots. About 87% of all strokes are the ischemic stroke. When someone has had a stroke and lived, it is usually an ischemic stroke, a stroke where an artery has been clogged by fatty deposits. When recovery begins after the stroke, it can take a long time because brain cells die immediately when they are deprived of oxygen. These brain cells never recover and the brain has to re-learn how to talk or how to move the parts of the body that were affected by the stroke. Again, like heart disease, atherosclerosis is the cause. Clogged arteries are the culprit. Atherosclerosis makes the arteries weak and susceptible to damage.

Chronic lower respiratory diseases comprise the fourth largest killer in America, which include asthma, emphysema and chronic bronchitis. What do your lungs have to do with blood viscosity? They're loaded with **blood vessels,** so just like heart and brains, lungs are highly vulnerable to the impact of poor circulation caused by saturated fats. Also, it's a known fact that asthma is associated with milk and cheese consumption, which sets up an allergic condition that makes lung problems worse by increasing mucus.

What do the four largest killers in America all have in common? **THEY ARE ALL DIRECTLY CAUSED BY, OR AGGREVATED BY, THE STANDARD AMERICAN DIET, SAD!**

It's pretty basic: clogged blood vessels set you up for disease in areas that need a constant blood supply. Of course we need a constant blood supply all throughout our bodies, but the fact is that certain, vital areas in the body require more blood supply than others, and the lack thereof causes a myriad of problems. Narrowing arteries cause heart attack, heart disease, stroke, lung problems, and diabetes, just to name a few. In fact, all the top killers in America come from food, saturated fats and the resulting clogged arteries! But there's more to the story than clogged arteries. A lot more.

The Kiso Diet™, in my opinion, is the best diet on the face of the planet for the majority of people. Why is it the best diet for most? Because, of what it's lacking! The reduction of saturated fat and animal protein is what's going to keep you younger inside and looking younger on the outside.

Chapter 4

Blood Thickness and the Kiso Diet™

Blood Viscosity

Why does blood tend to "stick" to the artery walls and narrow the passage way for oxygen to get through? **Blood thickness!** That's why!

FOODS YOU EAT CAUSE THE VISCOSITY OF YOUR BLOOD TO CHANGE!

When you eat a high fat diet (namely dairy products, red meats and eggs) your blood becomes sticky. Your blood becomes thick and sluggish! The viscosity of your blood goes up, meaning the fluidity of your blood goes down. This means that your heart has a harder time trying to "**push**" the blood throughout the body. Thick and sluggish blood causes your *blood pressure* to become higher.

Looking at this issue a little more closely, we need to understand a bit of how our bodies work. Your blood is composed of a symphony of life sustaining and health maintaining **particles**.

One of the better-known particles in your blood is the **red blood cell**. The red blood cell is shaped like a donut with a thin center. They are designed this way to deliver oxygen from your lungs to your tissues. In order to do this, the red blood cell must be maximally flexible and have the greatest amount of surface area possible through which to release its **oxygen molecules** at the right place. This is done through our arterial system; our larger blood vessels are called *arteries* and smaller ones called *arterioles.*

Another constituent of blood that "thickens" when eating "bad" foods are your *platelets.* **Platelets** are a big part of your blood, they are what's activated when you cut yourself. When your body has a cut, the body signals a blood clot to form so that the blood will stop leaking. *Platelet aggregation* takes place. In other words, the platelets, through a chemical process, change *fibrinogen* to *fibrin*, which makes the platelets stick together in order to clot the blood. When eating high amounts of SATURATED FATS, the platelets become "sticky" and slow the blood down, similar to when your body uses platelet aggregation to stop a blood vessel from leaking.

More information on what affects food has on blood viscosity...

Let's look more closely at the mechanism of why platelets get stickier with a bad diet. Eating lots of dietary fats causes platelet stickiness. Hormone-like substances called prostaglandins, derived from fatty acids in the blood, make the body produce prostacyclin, this is produced by cells in the blood vessel wall. Also, prostaglandins make the platelets produce thromboxane. Prostacyclin is what controls the muscular contraction of the blood vessel walls and prevents platelets from adhering. Thromboxane produced from the platelets determines the stickiness of the platelets and tends to cause the vessels to contract.

Prostaglandins differ in type depending on the type of fatty acids available. If lots of fatty acids (from animal protein, dairy foods, or eggs) are eaten, then Prostaglandin H2 (PGH2) is formed and the resultant thromboxane (TXA2) makes the platelets sticky. On the other hand, if lots of omega-rich, cold water fish and complex carbohydrates are eaten, then PGH3 and TXA3 are formed, and the platelets will be normal and not sticky. This positive effect is also seen when folks eat garlic and onions. That's why eating garlic and onions are key in the Kiso Diet™. Also taking Omega 3s or eating fish is not only allowed in the flexitarian portion of the Kiso Diet™, it's encouraged!

In large arteries, like the aorta that goes from your heart down in front of your spine, the blood vessels soar with blood. The arteries are huge, but in other areas of the body the areas are comprised of tiny little arterioles, which are so small that a red blood cell must bend in half to fit through them. Because of the red blood cell's unique shape it can fit through arterioles smaller than half its size. To get a proper picture of how small a red blood cell is, you can fit 5 million on top of a pinhead!

If your red blood cells are *sticky* or your blood is *thick* the cells begin to stick together. This not only decreases the amount of surface area through which your red blood cells can release oxygen, but two, three or more red blood cells clumped together prevent the single cell from bending over to pass through the smaller arterioles.

The result is that certain tissues do not get enough oxygen. When this occurs, the body, through a complex process of chemical and neurological messages, signals the heart to *pump harder.* This is one of the major causes of **high blood pressure.** There are other, more temporary, causes of high blood pressure such as dehydration or not drinking enough water or eating too much salt, but the biggest reason for *chronic* high blood pressure is eating lots of **saturated fats and animal protein.**

The viscosity of blood can be tested, and monitored. *Blood sedimentation rate* or **ESR** (erythrocyte sedimentation rate) can be used to determine *blood thickness.* It's a blood test that allows the blood to settle on the bottom of a test tube. The faster the blood settles the "sicker" your blood is. Blood settling quickly is a sign of illness. The blood's surface area is smaller and the blood cells fall like dinner plates piling on top of one another in clumps. Contrast this to healthy blood cells.

The healthy blood cells have a large surface area for carrying oxygen. Having a large surface area, the blood cells fall like snowflakes. They settle slowly, making the ESR longer *which is an indication of health.*

A blood test that shows blood viscosity is called the **PAT,** or *platelet adhesiveness (test) index.* The PAT test will show how slow or fast your blood clots. This test actually is a testament to how blood becomes sticky with poor diet. This test assesses the "stickiness" of the platelets. Dr Paul Owren, Hematologist at the Oslo University Hospital, devised a method of measuring platelet stickiness by means of observing the percentage of platelets that adhered to glass beads. The percentage is the index number. For example: A healthy young woman has a PAT number of 20 while a male with heart disease will have a number around 80. Also, any person who injures themselves regardless of their cardiovascular health will have a number around 90 for up to 15 days.

The PAT is a good test to use for determining if a person needs to adjust his or her diet. If a person's PAT index is consistently high, foods and nutrients can be taken to lower this number. Vitamin E, flaxseed oil, garlic, cod-liver oil, alcohol, lecithin and aspirin help.

Perhaps one of the reasons that French and Italian people living in those countries (not French or Italians living in

America because they tend to adopt the American life style) have less heart disease even though their diets are high fat, is because they are wine drinkers. Red wine has antioxidants called flavonoids (so does dark chocolate!) that have been shown to reduce atherosclerosis. There is one constituent called resveratrol, a type of flavonoid, which has been isolated and is said to be extremely powerful in reversing atherosclerosis or preventing atherosclerosis from happening. One can buy resveratrol from the health food store and take it as a supplement daily.

Also Omega 3s help combat atherosclerosis. One experiment illustrates the effectiveness of Omega 3s in lowering this number. Dr William Connor, Professor of Medicine, University of Oregon Clinical Nutrition Section, found that on a 10-day diet of salmon, patients' elevated cholesterol levels fell by 20% and triglycerides [fats] by 40-67%. These results are not entirely surprising because it has often been observed, but not before explained, that fishing communities in various parts of the world suffer a lower rate of heart attacks.

Have you ever heard of Linus Pauling? He had a theory about heart disease that was centered around lipoprotein, bad cholesterol (LDL) and the cardiovascular system. He wrote a book about how vitamin C could cure cancer, heart disease and a whole host of other things. He proposed that a deficiency of vitamin C resulted in the increased production of lipoprotein (LDL), which both hardened the arteries and caused blood clots. Here's how it works: Bad cholesterol or LDLs inhibit the breakdown of fibrin and fibrin makes blood viscosity go up or makes the blood thicker by making the platelets stickier. Lipoprotein (a form of LDL) is a key component in blood clot formation as well as increasing blood viscosity.

What lowers the bad cholesterol? Exercise and eating a low saturated fat diet as well as a diet low in animal proteins. As you will see later in this book, eating any type of animal protein, compared with vegetable sources of protein, can be a fertilizer for cancer. So it seems that not only is the saturated fat in meat detrimental to your health, but also the protein itself is not good if the protein circulates with "nothing to do." You've got to give the protein something to do, something to repair, then, magically, it's not the same threat that it was.

How do you give the protein something to do? Tear the body down a bit. Tearing the muscles increases your body's need for protein. Exercising increases your body's need for protein. Did you know that when Arnold Schwarzenegger built those 21 inch arms, he did that through a process of tearing the muscle down and letting the body build it back up better than it was before? Not only better, but stronger (not to mention bigger!) than it was before.

Some areas in the body are extremely susceptible to the thickening of blood. The prostate, for example. It often takes several months of antibiotics to get rid of a bacterial infection in the prostate. This is due to small arteries and veins that make it difficult for the antibiotic to get into the prostate with a high enough concentration to kill the pathogen. Logically, these tiny vessels also cause the prostate to be highly vulnerable to blood thickening.

Of course we know that blood thickening from eating bad foods can cause heart attack and stroke, but it can also cause more chronic conditions never really looked at before in any other diet book. I call high blood viscosity and what it causes, atherosclerosis, a **"holopathogenic" process. Holo** - means *whole* in Greek, **pathogenic** - means a *step-by-step development of a disease.*

This holopathogenic process hits virtually all areas of the body. Here are some areas of the body and the diseases that impact them, and it all starts from high blood viscosity.

1. Brain (Alzheimer's disease)

2. Thyroid (hyper/hypo thyroidism)

3. Kidneys (chronic kidney disease)

4. Prostate (infections/cancer)

5. Testicles and ovaries (cancer)

6. Joints of the body (degeneration/disc herniation)

I need to mention that areas in the body needing very *small arterioles* also need very *small veins*. Arteries and arterioles carry oxygenated blood from the heart to various areas in the body, while veins carry blood back to the heart. Also veins carry waste products from these areas, so if your blood is thick and greasy, or in other words, has high VISCOSITY then not only can't you get proper circulation into an area, but you cannot get proper blood flow out of an area. This means that not only would you have a *decreased amount of oxygen* in these key areas mentioned above, but also you would have a build-up of *toxins* and *waste* products in those areas. No wonder why so many people have problems in these key areas!

Prior to my research, I personally had never heard the connection of food related to so many areas of the body. That's why I've coined the word holopathogenic or holopathogenesis, because not only does atherosclerosis or a hardening or narrowing of the arteries affect the heart, it affects all of these other areas of the body as well.

Our medical science tends to segregate and breakdown everything into smaller and smaller details at the expense of looking at the *big picture.* Diagnosis is done this way. Our medical science is built upon diagnosing. The medical profession likes neat little categories that make it difficult for another physician to not know what the diagnosis means. By breaking things down or narrowing down the disease processes, it makes it easier for one physician to talk to another physician and for a physician to give a medicine for a particular disease. But the truth is that this disease process is **huge** and cannot be cured by one pill or 10 pills, it can only be cured by eating foods. *The right foods.*

Chapter 5

Joint Problems and Food

If you don't have good circulation, you don't have enough oxygenation in your tissues. We are not only talking about tissues of your brain and heart (stroke, heart disease), we are talking about other tissues, like your joints. Studies show the flow of blood is slowed considerably by a high fat diet. Fat clogs the system. It coats the red blood cells and platelets, and gets in the way of good clean circulation.

I'm a chiropractor, among other things. I've seen patients coming into my clinics for years with joint problems. Case in point. A 75 year-old patient comes into my clinic. He can barely walk due to swollen knees. He says his doctor told him he has arthritis and has lost the cartilage in his knee joints (both of them). We take x-rays of his lower back where he is now experiencing the most pain. His lower back is full of degeneration. It goes along with his knees. Well, he has widespread full-body degeneration; his spine, his shoulders, basically all over his body. This older man is an active bodybuilder. He lifts weights at least 4 times a week. I asked him about his diet and he says he has eaten meat all his life for protein. He wants to be big. He wants his muscles to be nicely developed so he eats a lot of protein in the form of red meat and pork.

I see this scenario all the time in my office: A heavy red meat eater with lots of degeneration throughout his body. He thought eating animal protein and drinking milk would help him retain his muscular size and in return, it's crippled him. He does have big muscles, even still at 75 years old, but he can barely walk.

Here's what happens when you eat lots of animal protein, and how eating excessive animal protein affects the joints.

All vertebrae in the body are joints. So not only are the ankles and shoulders and knees affected by eating excessive animal protein and saturated fat, but the vertebrae are affected as well. Being joints, joints in the human body have a characteristic. All these joints are made basically the same way. They have an airtight capsule surrounding them. Inside they have cartilage and on the surface of the joints, there are membranes that secrete a substance called synovial fluid. This fluid helps the joint glide when in use. Well, remember I mentioned earlier how the joints need circulation to survive? They are vascular, meaning they do have veins and arteries supplying blood, which gives the joints oxygen, and they do have a venous system that carries away the garbage. But, joints have a weird twist when it comes to their blood supply. Arteries and veins are not directly going into the joint. Oh no!

A network of arteries that look like a leaf covers the joints. Have you ever looked at a maple leaf and noticed how broad it is with veins running out from the center? That's similar to how your joints receive their blood supply. Each joint has an overlying "leaf," supplying indirect oxygen and nutrients, making it even more susceptible to atherosclerosis.

Here's what happens. Just like the heart that becomes choked off because of atherosclerosis and hardening of the arteries, your joints also suffer.

I noticed when I used to run a lot that my joints would hurt if I had eaten meat, or if I had drank a lot of milk, or had eaten some eggs before running. I correlated this finding years ago, before I was a doctor. Just like your heart, your joints lose their blood supply by being surrounded by thick blood. Blood that's filled with saturated fats and cholesterol. The blood, being thicker, does not penetrate the joints as well and the joint starts to suffer. Having a decreased blood supply to the joint, whether the joint is a knee joint, a shoulder joint or a vertebrae in your back, is going to make the joint painful. It suffers when you can't get enough blood to the joint itself.

I used to wonder why shoulder injuries in Japan were termed "goju-kata," meaning 50's shoulder. The average person in America or Japan starts to have vascular changes around the age of 50. That's when you usually start having prostate problems, heart problems and problems with your joints, as well as, not to mention, hemorrhoids. So in the joints, when there is a decreased blood supply, degeneration starts to set in! Joints, especially knees, can hurt right after eating a high fat meal. But the long-term effects of eating high fat meals, which go along with fatty animal protein, will definitely take their toll on the joints as years go by.

So, there it is my friends...the TRUTH about how to stay young inside and outside. Eat less mammalian animal fat, which goes along with eating less animal protein. ***DO NOT EAT MORE PROTEIN THAN YOUR BODY NEEDS ON A DAILY BASIS!***

Chapter 6

Blood flow and its implications...

Why did Yale University find that vegetarians had twice as much stamina compared to ATHLETES who were meat eaters? Only half the vegetarians worked out at all, the other half were completely sedentary! Why did they out perform the meat eaters (athletes!) in endurance? The vegetarians' blood was thinner, thinner blood performs better. It carries more oxygen and doesn't clog up the muscles, joints and lungs when you do exercise.

In Japan, there is a Taiko group called Tao. Taiko is a very rigorous traditional kind of drumming. They use heavy, thick drumsticks and pound hard and fast for extended periods of time. This Taiko group is one of the most famous drumming groups in Japan. They tour for 6 months at a time, once a year. When touring, they stay isolated in a mountain retreat in Kyushu Japan. They live together, eat together that way they can play together well, and play together they do! When touring, they ALL become vegetarian. They're not vegetarian when not touring, but become vegetarian while they are playing for about 6 months a year. Why? Because they claim that eating any meat of any kind slows them down. If one of them ate meat, that person would not be able to keep up with the others. It's interesting that they also say their sweat becomes sticky if they do eat meat and is a major problem when they play at events. They claim that their endurance is so affected by eating meat that even one meal of meat causes them to not have the endurance needed to complete one event! Their habits exemplify how meat slows down your blood flow...let's look at some other issues.

Knowing what you know... Let's look at the other diseases that devastate our American population.

Let's start with a hydraulic pump...

Why is Viagra such a top selling drug? Because since our country has the Standard American Diet, which stands for SAD, many American men have a problem with impotence, more medically termed: Erectile Dysfunction Syndrome. Another closely related topic is prostate trouble.

OK, women don't have prostates, lucky them, but most American men and women are following the SAD diet. Yes...they may not know it, but they ARE on a diet...the SAD diet! Remember, we eat culturally, without thinking, and it's sad that our SAD diet is part of OUR culture! With all that cholesterol clogging our veins and arteries, men start to experience prostate problems. These various prostate problems are said to come with age. But in unindustrialized nations, prostate problems are unheard of! What does this tell you?!

Here it is, straight from the horse's mouth (not quite, but I like citing the big institutions when it comes to statistics, that way everyone will believe me, ha-ha). The latest American Cancer Society estimates for prostate cancer in the United States are for 2010:

217,730 new cases of prostate cancer will be diagnosed.

32,050 men will die of prostate cancer.

1 man in 6 will be diagnosed with prostate cancer during his lifetime.

Sounds bleak? It is. But if you eat more fiber and less meat and dairy you will cure your prostate problems. Why do you think that cancer strikes the prostate? It's because it's a very vascular area in the body. In other words, it needs a strong blood supply. It needs constant blood flow. When areas in the body that require lots of blood flow get choked off from atherosclerosis, the result is ischemia, or lack of blood flow and lack of oxygen.

The body needs and depends on this blood flow to bring nutrients to these highly vascular areas and also to take waste products back through the vascular system. When this does not function, disease ensues. It may result in pain or prostate infections from opportunistic bacteria. Eventually it may lead to cancer. So not only will we see in this book that cancer is caused from excess animal proteins, but also that it is caused by a lack of arterial blood from atherosclerosis and plaque anywhere in the body. The body's healing ability is shackled when a lack of circulation is present in an area.

We can learn a lot by studying the *penis.* Essentially, the penis is a **hydraulic pump**, highly vascular. It has characteristics that are unlike anything else in the body and it's great for using it as an example of how the body is affected by thick blood. *According to a JAMA (a popular medical journal) study,* **45 percent** *of those who have erectile dysfunction end up having a* **stroke or heart attack***. Now do ya believe me?*

Well, if you have erectile dysfunction syndrome you can bet that it's caused from a lack of blood flow to the penis. Why do we get a lack of blood flow in areas of the body? Thick, viscous blood and atherosclerosis! What does Viagra do? The well-known blue pill that makes you have an erection when you may not have had an erection for years? It opens up the arteries around the penis. All of a sudden, an erection happens. You can bet if a pill can open your arteries, it's also opening up blood vessels, not only in your penis, but in other areas of your body as well! This could be dangerous for some people. The point is, opening up the blood flow to the penis helps a person have an erection. Well, if you are eatin' lots of animal proteins, drinking milk, eating dairy products and eating lots of eggs, your penis suffers just like the rest of your body. The cure...START EATING LESS OF THOSE THINGS or NONE OF THOSE THINGS until you "cure" yourself of this problem. Once you cure yourself from this problem, I guarantee that you will watch what you eat from then on!

What happens to the penis happens to the rest of your body!

Here's a statistic for you. During a man's reproductive years, regular meat eating will lower sperm count, shorten sperm life, decrease ejaculate volume, and cause infertility. All of these problems are largely absent in those who abstain from meat, dairy and eggs. The same arterial system that's too clogged to send blood to the penis is also slowly but surely becoming too clogged to send blood to the brain and heart.

Why is this happening? Erectile dysfunction is usually seen in men with high cholesterol levels and high levels of LDL "bad" cholesterol. Both of those conditions are brought on by regular meat consumption. You eat the fatty stuff, it layers your arteries, and blood flow is decreased. Simple as that. Looking at it another way, the plot thickens!! Or, more accurately, the blood thickens!

Chapter 7

Milk, Milk Protein and Animal Protein

cause CANCER

Cancer and a plant-based diet...

For those who are looking for a "cure" for cancer, don't ask the AMA (American Medical Association) or even the American Cancer Society. They only use "conventional" means to fight cancer. Conventional ways are chemotherapy and radiation along with surgery. Chemotherapy and radiation are dangerous and devastating for your immune system. Often times, after going through all of these procedures, the cancer returns. Why? Because they did not address the issue of WHY the cancer came in the first place. For many, chemo saved their lives, but the reason "why" they got cancer was not addressed at all...their diet.

What causes cancer

There is a book that will blow your socks off called **The China Study**. It was written by T. Colin Campbell Ph.D. This book was written about a study done by Cornell University and Oxford University, examining 65 countries in rural China back in the 1970s, 1980s, and early 1990s.

The author started out believing that cancer could be cured by protein. As he researched this position, he found the opposite was true. Injecting rats with a carcinogen (cancer causing substance), all the rats became infected with liver cancer. When he gave the rats a 20% protein diet, 100% of the rats died. When he gave the rats a 5% protein diet, 100% of the rats lived. The more protein he gave the rats, the faster the rats died. From this study, they found that a plant-based, vegetarian diet low in protein, cured cancer better than any regime of cancer fighting procedures we currently now possess.

In the wake of these findings, many cancer-curing establishments formed within the United States. These centers focused their attention on using a plant-based diet to not only cure cancer but a whole other host of diseases, such as diabetes, gout, arthritis, multiple sclerosis, and lupus, just to name a few. For example, these natural "cure" centers were curing type II diabetes in five to six days! I know it sounds amazing, but it's true. The list of cancers cured by these natural centers is massive. These centers largely moved out of the United States to nearby Mexico to escape the wrath of the United States government and the AMA and FDA. The government makes a lot of money "fighting" cancer and there is no money in fighting cancer for the American Medical Association or the American Cancer Society, using *natural therapies*.

Basically here is the skinny on cancer...

We have cancer cells in our bodies everyday. Our immune system kills them immediately. Only 5% of actual cancer comes from carcinogens in the "environment," the rest comes from diet, genetics and a low immune system. Many cancers return or move into other areas of the body because the individual's body is allowing the cancer to reside in their body.

These cancer cells that we have in our bodies that are usually killed by our immune system, are "seeds." Some of these seeds are planted in our bodies by carcinogens in the environment (about 5%). However, most of these seeds are planted by foods that we take into our bodies. According to the China Study about 93% of all cancers come from diet. Only 3% are estimated to come from genetics. That's why natural cancer and wellness centers concentrate on diet first.

What is the biggest cancer fertilizer in foods? **Animal protein**! It's animal protein that causes the seeds to grow; it's like fertilizer. Animal protein fertilizes the cancer seeds to grow. So if you eliminate or sharply reduce animal protein in your diet, your chances of getting cancer are sharply reduced.

Animal protein is also the cause of many other diseases that strike many Americans. Diseases like stroke, diabetes, and heart disease. This is mostly due to red meats (or *mammalian meats,* as I like to call them) having lots of cholesterol and lots of saturated fats.

Corporations and big business influence what we hear from the media...

Why isn't this knowledge about cancer talked about in every home, not only in America, but across the globe? The reason for this is because it's bad business for the world's largest corporations. Meat and meat products sell and make big money!

Listen to this. If you're old enough, do you remember the hot dog scare, or nitrite scare, of the early seventies? We heard that hot dogs and lunch meats having nitrites put in them to enhance color and taste were linked to cancer in rats. Yes, I remember. I heard people say, "You don't want to eat hot dogs now." Then, again in 1979, Ralph Nader said that hot dogs were "deadly missiles." Wow, that statement turned a few heads (away from their hot dogs!).

Well after the hoopla, the government told companies involved with nitrites to not put so much in the products and the issue went away. You know what caused Ralph to say such a thing? It was because over 10% of laboratory rats died after being fed nitrites, a lot of nitrites, instead of just over 5% of them dying from cancer naturally. This 5% increase stirred up America.

Can you imagine what this new information from the China Study would do if it was widely heard? The information that you could *turn off cancer and turn it back on* again **like a light switch**, **100% of the time**, by not eating or eating animal protein? Corporations and the news media don't want this information in your knowledge base. If everyone knew and believed it, it would definitely change the way Americans eat.

Cancer "cure" centers...

At these wellness centers, eating a plant-based diet without any animal protein (that means no meat of any kind or dairy for that matter), cures not only heart disease and diabetes but also cures auto immune diseases like rheumatoid arthritis, multiple sclerosis, and lupus.

So in my mind, when I think of longevity and living healthy, being vegetarian is the number one method (tho we'll see that eating fish ain't bad either). Also in the China Study, they found that the worst animal proteins, those that fertilized cancer seeds the most, were the proteins from milk and dairy! It was **casein protein** that got the nod for the worst protein you could eat for fertilizing cancer cells to grow. Milk does a body good? Not unless you're a baby cow!

Casein is found in milk, cheese and yogurt, from all the animals in the world (80 to 85% of milk protein is casein protein). "Milk does a body good," the old campaign from the Milk Advisory Board, makes it sound like cow's milk is the perfect thing to ingest for a healthy body - NOT. As humans, we can digest milk when we are young because of an enzyme called lactase. Between the ages of 18 months and 24 months, we lose the ability to digest milk protein because we gradually lose 95% of this enzyme. After that, we cannot fully digest the milk we consume and because of the acidic nature of undigested milk, we get a build up of bad bacteria in the gut. To varying degrees, all humans become lactose intolerant. This is why, if you have irritable bowel syndrome or have diverticulitis, drinking milk is a risky proposition.

How about milk and calcium? We've all heard that milk gives you calcium for strong bones and helps you avoid osteoporosis. This, in fact, is just not true. Listen to this. A study 12-year study of 78,000 women found **no evidence** that drinking milk helped reduce osteoporosis and hip fracture. In fact, they found that women who drank more than two glasses per day had a 1.5 times higher risk of hip fracture compared with women who only drank one glass of milk a week or less!

According to the Bowes and Church's food values of portions commonly used, milk may have 300mg of calcium, but only 32% of that is actually absorbed! You can derive this much from 1 ½ cups of broccoli.

Another problem with milk consumption is the protein in milk, it has lots of protein. The proteins in milk cause acid. This acid has to be buffered by your body. One of the things your body uses to buffer acid in your blood is calcium, taken from your bones! That's why, I believe, the study cited showed that women who drank only one cup of milk a week, or less, had less hip fractures than women who drank two glasses of milk daily. Even the FDA says that there is no evidence that milk helps with osteoporosis or hip fractures.

Do ya believe me now? You don't need the stuff. I had a patient tell me that she's on the milk diet. I asked her, "What's the milk diet?" She said, "The casein protein in milk can't be absorbed completely, so it curdles in your stomach and it makes you not want to eat for long periods of time and ya don't get hungry so I can lose weight!" That's amazing, using the indigestibility of milk to help you lose weight. But I checked it out and it's true. Casein protein in milk, besides fertilizing cancer, curdles in your stomach and causes indigestion and a sense of being full. People do use this method to lose weight! Not smart.

How about lactose intolerance? People can be lactose intolerant and really not know it. Did you know that 90 to 100% of Asians are lactose intolerant? Native Americans are 95% lactose intolerant. Even Italians and African Americans are between 65-75 lactose intolerant. Lactose intolerance causes milk proteins to not be absorbed properly, this causes a condition known as leaky gut syndrome. This syndrome has been linked to rheumatoid arthritis and multiple sclerosis. People have all kinds of allergies to milk, cheese and eggs but they just keep on eating and drinking it despite their inability to stop their sinus headaches and runny noses. They say, "Well, I'm allergic to dust" or pollen or a whole host of other things. Let me tell you that the allergies you develop to milk can make your body's immune system run amok. You've excited your immune system with constant allergic reactions first stemming from milk, and then your body becomes so sensitive that now you're allergic to weeds, dust mites, flowers and blue sky!

There is a wonderful landmark book called ***Diet for a New America,*** written by John Robbins, son of Irv Robbins, famous founder of the ice cream shop Baskin Robbins. John is a vegan and would not personally drink milk or eat ice-cream (after he became an adult). In his book, he writes about vegetarianism as well as the harmfulness of milk. Great book! He even states that if Americans ate just 10% less meat, the crops not fed to animals to produce meat would allow everyone in the world to have enough food to eat! That's amazing! The industrialized cattle industry, which includes milk, destroys the land. You can find more information about this book at www.earthsave.org.

Now, on to the nitty-gritty…

Chapter 8

Protein

Protein is essential for life and the repair of the body. But getting too much protein in animal form is the root of promoting cancer in our bodies. It's said that each person actually has six to seven bouts of serious cancer in one's lifetime. I first heard this watching a movie entitled "Healing Cancer from the inside," by Mike Anerson.

Dr. T. Colin Campbell Ph.D, was featured in the movie and inspired me to buy his book, **The China Study** (mentioned in the last chapter). I used the book in my nutrition class at the Traditional Chinese Medical College of Hawaii, a master's degree course in oriental medicine. My class went bonkers over the book, many students bought the book for family members on the mainland.

The book was an account of Dr. Campbell's findings that he logged over a 25 year period studying diet in and around rural China. His findings changed his own eating habits. He was raised on a farm and when he started the China study he thought that protein would be the one thing that would *"change the world and end disease."* He thought that protein would be the *"cure all"* for cancer.

When he was in the Philippines studying a carcinogen called Aflotoxin and it's relationship to liver cancer, he heard the details of an experiment performed in India, the results of which were very interesting to him. The experiment showed that **protein actually "caused"** cancer.

After his stint in the Philippines was over, Dr. Campbell got a grant to study diet in rural China while he was employed as a professor at *Cornell University*. He was able to actually perform his own experiments on protein and found the exact same results as the experiment done earlier in India. He found that when rats were given animal protein, in the amount of 20 percent of their total daily dietary intake of calories, 100 percent of the rats died. When he gave rats an animal protein diet of 5 percent of their total daily dietary intake of calories, 100 percent of the rats lived! Wow, yes, black and white. Who ever thought that eating protein would *kill you*.

As we now know, he later found that *casein protein* was the worst protein for "promoting" cancer. This is what was fed to the rats during the experiment. He also found that this "promotion" of cancer did not occur with *plant-based proteins,* for example, *soy protein.*

Why do I say "promoting"? Dr. Campbell found out that animal protein was the culprit for fertilizing (promoting) cancer to grow. More importantly, **casein protein,** which comprises 80% to 85% of all the protein in milk, was found not to initiate cancer but to promote cancer.

When we get what's known as a foci or a spot of cancer, that foci of cancer can quickly become a tumor of cancer. This foci is essentially a seed. What promotes this foci to grow into a tumor is animal protein. Yes folks, eating a diet low in animal protein can save your life.

Many types of cancers, like skin cancer, are so directly related to the promotion by animal proteins that in the movie, "Healing cancer from the inside," they state that "skin cancer can be completely controlled by the amount and kind of protein we eat." Either the cancer can be shut off by eating low amounts of animal protein or eating plant protein, or turned on by eating a *large amount of animal protein.*

In fact, Dr. Campbell describes in his book **The China Study** that he found, with amazement, that cancer could be turned on and off again depending on how much the subject ate in the way of animal proteins. He also found that eating protein from vegetable sources did not promote cancer in any way.

Meats

If you love meat, eat it sparingly, combining it correctly so you don't develop an upset stomach. (If you eat meat with lots of carbohydrates, it can upset your stomach making digestion difficult. Eating it with rice or potatoes is for some, OK.) Or, try eating only chicken and different fowls. Remember, red meat is a mammalian source of meat. It causes high blood viscosity because of its inherent high cholesterol and saturated fats.

I've often thought that red meats, coming from mammals, are **too close** to our own mammalian bodies, and if we eat them, it harms our own bodies. Who knows, maybe **it's almost like the cannibal thing, you know, it's not right to eat your own species!**

If you must, steaks should be eaten only occasionally, because even a lean steak is still about 60% fat! Look at it this way, YOU ARE ONE HUGE FILTER! That's right, you take things in: water, salts, food, oils, and then must process them through your body. Imagine the grease found in one steak caught in a filter. Yes, your body has to filter that steak too and the grease sticks to things like your digestive tract and arteries! Just keep this in mind.

Hormones in the meat...

If you do choose to eat meat, it's really important to buy only organic meat. The biggest problem with regular, non-organic meats are the hormones present in the meat products. Did you ever watch a movie filmed in the 1940's?

People walking around were bone thin. Now, look at the people in movies walking around. They are huge! I say it's not all because of FAT you know, it's also because of HORMONES!

The cattle and chicken industries put hormones into their animals to make them bigger and fatter. The bigger and fatter they are, the more money they bring. Also, the FASTER they become big and fat, the faster the money comes in.

I saw a movie you may have seen called FOOD INC. (A very good movie by the way.) When I saw the inside of a chicken factory, I noticed that all the chicken torsos were the same size! It was amazing! How were they all the same size? The reason...Because these chickens were given the same amount of hormones and their bodies grew at the same rate, then they were slaughtered at the same time. In fact, their bodies grew so fast that the chickens could not stand. Plus, almost all these chickens were raised in the dark. What's wrong with this picture? HELLO!

Hormones found in meat are a hidden bomb often overlooked by people buying meat and meat products. These hormones are especially dangerous for children, as their small bodies are especially vulnerable to antibiotic and hormone residues.

In the U.S., most farmers (80%) continue to administer powerful growth-stimulating steroids to cattle and antibiotics to all animals raised for food. The antibiotics are necessary to keep the animals alive in the un-healthful environments in which they're raised until they're old enough to be slaughtered.

I have noticed recently that big chain supermarkets are starting to carry meats that have "no hormones" written on the package. Very good! Now, listen to this! The Cancer Prevention Coalition warns, "No dietary levels of hormones are safe, and a dime-sized piece of meat contains billions of millions of [hormone] molecules." That's scary! Hormones in meat, especially dairy cows and beef, are blamed for the early sexual development of young girls in the U.S. Nearly half of all African-American girls and about 15 percent of Caucasian American girls now go into puberty when they are just eight years old.

According to the European Union's Scientific Committee, the meat industry uses six growth hormones in beef production. These six hormones include three that are naturally occurring—Oestradiol, Progesterone and Testosterone—and three that are synthetic, which are Zeranol, Trenbolone, and Melengestrol. These hormones have been proven to disrupt the hormone balance in *our* bodies. They also have been found to cause developmental problems in children, interfering with the reproductive system in adolescents and adults, and even leading to the development of breast, prostate or colon cancers. If you ingest female hormones from meat, you will get more "female" hormone. As a woman, the more estrogen you eat, the higher the incidence of breast cancer. After all this, guess what? The hormone residue in cow feces gets into our ground water and a whole other problem arises. Wide spread contamination of our lands! It's all scary. That's why it's so important to shop at the health food stores. Animals bound for health food stores are raised more humanely and more healthfully, for them and for us.

Moral of the story...**Don't eat non-organic meat!** In China where their blood marker (we'll talk about blood markers later) for heart disease is lower, they eat fewer animals than we do. Their incidence of breast cancer is 1/5 that compared with the United States. **Listen people!**

One more thing, it's a consciousness thing...

When studying disciplines like Yoga or meditation, many people become vegetarian because it is claimed that your "balance" is better, meaning you are less hot tempered or you can concentrate on spiritual things to a greater extent. This may be due to the fact that it is said that we receive "hormones of rage" when we eat animals. Animals feel the stress of being slaughtered and this creates "bad" hormones and substances like adrenalin and cortisol. Also animals that are not properly cared for during their lifetime before being slaughtered are filled with the "chemicals of suffering." These substances are passed from their bodies to our bodies through meat consumption, and can influence our behavior. So it's something to consider.

You might start at stage three (after your initiation period) in the Kiso Diet™ initially and move into being a vegetarian as time goes on. Also as one gets older, over 50 years of age or so, in the orient, many people eat more vegetarian as their age progresses and their digestive systems get more sensitive.

Ever heard of **Rudolf Steiner**? He created the Woldorf educational system, and says that "eating animal protein clogs up the *etheric body*" of our auric system. So our arteries are not the only thing that gets clogged up eating excess animal protein, your *spiritual energy system* also suffers...**so within...so without!**

How good is vegetable protein compared with animal protein? Good question. Dr. Campbell found that eating only vegetable protein would not promote cancer at all. In fact eating only "plant source" proteins and a total vegan diet reversed cancer. That's why cancer "cure" centers around the world like The Healing Oasis with Dr. Lodi, M.D. and Brenda

Cobb founder of The Living Foods Institute in Atlanta Georgia, only use vegan sources for food.

It's true that you need several sources of plant-based protein to equal animal protein. This can be accomplished simply with proper food combining. For example, eating beans with bread. The two foods complement each other because **vegetable protein lacks certain essential amino acids,** but these are present in bread and rice thus forming a meal with a complete protein source.

I often have people ask me about plant protein supplements. If you are going to supplement your body with any protein, I recommend a plant-based protein supplement for obvious reasons. However, if you are a person lifting weights and want to add muscle and you want an animal source of protein, I suggest whey or egg protein.

Stay away from any kind of casein protein, remember, casein protein is the biggest cancer promoter. Also, keep this in mind, just supplement once or twice a day with no more than 15 to 20 grams of protein at a time. The reason...your kidneys. Your kidneys don't do well when you overload them with protein. Remember I said YOU are like a big filter, well, your kidneys are the master filters of your body. Protein can "clog" up your kidneys and make your kidneys ache and hurt. If this happens, you'll feel an ache in the lower mid back around the kidney area. The other problem with protein powders is the incidence of intestinal obstruction. That's why I recommend not taking too much protein at a whack.

Now, the **best protein source for protein powder for building muscle is... whey or egg.** After this, we have the plant-based proteins. There are different sources like spirulina, and hemp, but **soy** gets the nod for being the most complete protein. Soy protein does not have all the essential amino acids to be a "complete" protein like whey and eggs, it's just slightly off. But manufacturers of soy protein powders have put in the few *missing links* to make it a **whole protein**. Soy has some *phytoestrogens* (female hormones), so men should not take a ton. How about women? I'll discuss that next.

There is a measurement of how effective proteins are in the human body, it's called PDCAAS (Protein Digestibility Corrected Amino Acid Score). Whey leads the list. There is another measurement, it's called **BV (biological value)**. BV is just another scale on which to judge the nutritional value of proteins, and is more widely used.

Here are the figures for some of the top proteins using BV for the numbers. Whey proteins again lead this table, with a score of 104, leaving behind all other sources of proteins, such as eggs (100), **soy proteins (74),** peanuts (68), and wheat proteins (54). But as I said earlier, some other plant-based proteins are added to soy, to make it more effective.

How about the BV for different animal meats? Eggs are 100, **fish is 83**, beef and cheese are 80, and chicken is 79. That's why eating pesco vegetarian (vegetarian plus fish) is great (except for the toxins in fish). As a vegetarian, eating some eggs (only 3 eggs a week!), soy, beans, and cheese (for flavor), you can get plenty of protein.

What about soy anyway...

Soy protein is very popular among vegetarians. Soy proteins are especially effective for women with hormonal imbalances, and help with post-menopausal problems. Infants and kids can eat soybeans to help in the growth of the body. Vitamin B_{12}, a substance found in animal protein, is *abundantly found* in soybeans so it's the best natural option for vegetarians.

Is soy all good?...Yes, pretty much. A lot of stuff has been said recently about soy *phytoestrogens.* They may cause breast cancer etc. Much of this propaganda about how bad soy is was done by soy's adversary...**the milk people**! I read this in John Robbins' book, *The Food Revolution*. In this book, John points out that the Milk Advisory Board views soy as a genuine threat to its industry.

Dietary estrogen (phytoestrogen) can be found in foods, oils and herbs. Below is a short list of phytoestrogen food sources analyzed by researchers in Canada. This Canadian research team found out the amounts of these phytoestrogens in various foods, oils and herbs.

Total phytoestrogen content presented below is the sum of isoflavones (genistein, daidzein, glycitein, formononetin), lignans (secoisolariciresinol, matairesinol, pinoresinol, lariciresinol), and coumestan (coumestrol).

Food sources	Phytoestrogen content(µg/100g)
Flax seed	379380
Soybeans	103920
Tofu	27150.1
Soy yogurt	10275
Sesame seed	8008.1
Flax bread	7540
Multigrain bread	4798.7
Soymilk	2957.2
Hummus	993
Garlic	603.6
Mungbean sprouts	495.1
Dried apricots	444.5
Alfalfa sprouts	441.4

Dried dates	329.5
Sunflower seed	216
Chestnuts	210.2
Olive oil	180.7
Almonds	131.1
Green bean	105.8
Peanuts	34.5
Onion	32
Blueberry	17.5
Corn	9
Coffee, regular	6.3
Watermelon	2.9
Milk, cow	1.2

As you can see, flax seeds, soybeans and tofu are up at the top with high counts of phytoestrogens. These phyto-estrogens are not exactly hormones, but they are close and can "trick" the body a bit. For example, Japanese women have a very light menopause. Their pre and post menopausal symptoms are much less than that of American women. Why? Because they eat and drink more soy, tofu and miso compared with Americans. They even love to eat something called Nato or decayed soybeans! Very stinky stuff, but very good for the body and digestive system! Many say that once you get used to the taste, you can't stop eating it as a snack! I once had a young Japanese woman work in one of my clinics. She had the strangest boyfriend. I finally asked her, "why did you pick a boyfriend like him?" She said, "He's like nato, once you get used to it, you can't live without it!" Very funny!

If you are a man and drink an excessive amount of soymilk (over 2 cups a day), you can start to have a reduced sex drive, reduced facial hair, nipple contractions and other feminizing qualities because soy's phytoestrogens are very close to estrogen. (Since it's NOT estrogen, it does not promote breast cancer like regular hormonal estrogen). Those symptoms sound like a good reason to avoid soy, but there are MANY, MANY health benefits from soy consumption. For instance, drinking just one to two glasses of soymilk a day reduces the incidence of prostate cancer in men by 70%.

Studies done on the effects of phytoestrogens on men don't show a huge change in the blood work of these men. Women, on the other hand, are influenced to a much greater extent than men. This is a good thing in my opinion. I don't think there's any need for concern for men or women about health risks from eating soy. Just exercise a little caution with drinking soymilk. While its phytoestrogen count isn't as high as dietary soy (like tofu), the average serving of soymilk is larger than the usual serving of dietary soy. So eat as much dietary soy as you like, but limit your soymilk consumption to two glasses a day.

I do have a funny but true story concerning my own experiences with soymilk. In the late 90s I used to go to Trader Joe's and load up on soymilk. Soymilk had become pretty popular and I loved it. I used to load my cart up with soymilk and, at the time allergic to cow's milk, I drank a ton. Well, one day getting out of the shower, I looked in the mirror and noticed that my nipples had turned white. My wife was standing nearby and saw them and said "what's wrong with your nipples?" I said "I don't know." After checking out the situation, I realized that my nipples were so contracted that they were experiencing a lack of blood flow.

It was then that I started to investigate the downside of soymilk; too much phytoestrogen packed in every cup. I was having nipple contractions! Wow, this was not only hilarious but shocking! I took myself totally off soymilk and to my surprise, it took about three months for the phenomenon to go away. Well, during the time I stayed away from t-shirts and sheer nighties!

Chapter 9

Our Gas Tanks…

Carbohydrates…

Some diets, for example, the low carb diets like the Atkins Diet and the South Beach Diet, shun carbs. If you shun carbs what else are you supposed to eat? Well, in the Atkins Diet, you eat fats and proteins. Burning these two fuels for energy puts the body in crisis. Does it make you lose weight? Yes, it can do a very good job of helping you lose weight at the expense of your health. The South Beach Diet takes it easy on fats compared to the Atkins Diet and allows more carbohydrates, but you can still have some problems. Basically, if you only eat proteins and fat, then your body is forced to burn fat using a process called ketosis.

So what? You ask… Let's introduce the gas tank concept, with food as our fuel.

Our bodies have three gas tanks, each with its own function, all there to help us. The carbohydrate tank is the largest. Then there is the fat tank. Last is the protein tank, which is quite small. When our bodies run off of the fuel in these tanks, the waste each produces is quite different. Also the process the body uses to burn these fuels is quite different.

Carbohydrates are the easiest fuel for our bodies to convert into energy, so the fuel in the carb tank is what we burn first. When we temporarily run out of carbs, we can burn fats and proteins but something happens on the way to the farm. Acid is created! Lots of acid in the body creates a condition called acidosis. That's why folks on the Atkins Diet start to have bad breath. The acidity in the body comes out in the breath and through your kidneys. That's also why people on the Atkins Diet have had kidney problems as well as kidney failure, which often ends up with those folks dying.

Yes, our protein tank is small and small for a reason. Protein is stored in our bodies in the form of muscle. It's not ideal to "burn" up our muscles and connective tissue in order for our bodies to stay alive, but it's a defense mechanism of our bodies for this to happen under extreme duress, but only in times of starvation. We saw this in pictures of the prisoners in World War II at Auschwitz. As the body wastes away under starvation, fat is used first, then the body tries to use the muscles for fuel to stay alive. Let me let you in on a little secret...WE ARE MEANT TO RUN ON CARBOHYDRATES!

Yes, it's true, we are meant to run on carbs. Just look at the history of human beings on this planet for the past 100,000 thousand years. We have been hunters, farmers, fisherman, you name it, we've been it. But throughout history, man did not eat protein alone. Until very recently, man ate a largely plant-based diet supplemented with occasional animal protein.

Early man did not go to the gym, work out his biceps and go home to the couch and let the protein eaten sink into his muscles so he would look better at the beach! Early man walked a lot, moving to find more game, moving to avoid bad weather. Along the way, they ate carbohydrates in the form of fruits, vegetables and grains found in their areas.

How about the fat gas tank? Glad you asked. When we eat fat, that fat is sometimes burned for fuel before it makes it to the storage tank. Fat is a pretty good source of energy actually. If we had a glass of milk and a hamburger for lunch, our body, in its wisdom, burns some of the fat eaten for fuel. But most of it is stored in our fat tanks (called fat cells) to hopefully be used at a later time, like, for instance, in case one needs extra fuel on the way around the mountain range in 40,000 B.C. Oh yes, or when you skip a meal because you had to work through lunch because of that damn virus that hacked into your computer this morning. Your body is more adept at burning fat than protein. But the byproduct of burning fat...again is acid. Not something you want to live on for long periods of time. Again, burning stored fat is a defense mechanism our bodies use under times of duress, just not as drastic as the protein burning defense mechanism. So for those who leave out carbs and eat fat and protein to burn protein and fat stores in your body, go ahead, but at best, it's dangerous.

Are you wondering how a low carb diet makes you lose weight? When you eat carbohydrates in large amounts, it raises your blood's glucose level, which raises the blood's insulin level. Insulin does two things: it makes your body store the fat you eat in your fat stores and then it shuts the door on the releasing of fat from these fat stores. So the low carb diets use this technology to lose weight. Because eating fat and protein does not activate glucose, the body is able to release fat from the fat cells, without storing new fat into those fat cells. So what does the body do? It burns the fat in your body.

Following a low carb diet allows you to eat anything you want, even fatty foods, because the body does not store fat on account of the body not releasing insulin. So, since there are no carbs to use as fuel (or very little), the body burns fat, both stored fat and the fat you just ate. Yes, it works as a weight loss method. BUT the downside is...acid. The low carb diets are called ketogenic diets. Ketones are acid molecules and are generated as the body burns fat. When we burn fat, ATP is created which is a source of energy, but the down side is that ketones are also created. There is one type of ketone that is created called acetone. Acetone must be secreted in the urine and the breath. A condition called ketoacidosis can develop which can be life threatening for some individuals. So that's how the low carb diet works. Come on, think about it. Eating high fat and protein and losing weight? At the expense of your health? Not for me!

Back to the carbohydrate gas tank. Oh yes, the carbohydrate gas tank is big. It's the one we are SUPPOSED TO USE! It's the cleanest burning one. It's like comparing Diesel fuel (protein) and regular gasoline fuel (fat) with propane (carbohydrate). The diesel smells, regular gas also smells but not as bad as diesel. But propane is great, it's much cleaner. It's also better for the environment. No, carbohydrate's waste is not exactly like propane's, but now I'll bet you'll remember this analogy. My point is, the waste products and the processes the body uses to burn carbohydrates is the BEST for your body. It's the one we were meant to burn on a day-to-day basis. Now even the FDA is saying, yeah, you should eat about 65% of all your foods in the form of carbohydrates. Ah, but not all carbohydrates are the same... Read on...

We have complex carbs and simple carbs. Complex carbs, of all the carbohydrates, are what we want to eat 90% of the time. Why only 90%? Because the other 10% are tasty and fun to eat and allow you to enjoy all the complexities of having a good and enjoyable diet.

Complex carbs are carbohydrates that have been taken out of nature as whole foods. This means they have been taken out of their environment as whole items. For example: Brown rice is a great carbohydrate. The rice grains have been removed from the plant, but still have the husk, the covering that makes it "brown". It is still whole. When we eat brown rice it give us not only nutrition and energy, it also gives us fiber. That's the way "whole foods" are. Being whole they possess all kinds of good qualities. They are a great source of energy, vitamins and minerals as well as giving us fiber.

What are simple carbs? Simple carbs are carbohydrates taken out of nature and "denatured" or refined. Refining means taking this once natural carbohydrate and stripping it of most of its original natural form to use some part of it. For example, taking a wheat straw, then peeling away all the whole parts to make wheat flour. It's not so bad if we stop there, but when we add bleach to further break it down into mostly sugar and give it that fluffy, doughy taste we came to love eating white bread as a kid, there's very little left of the original nutrients. Our tongues got used to certain tastes when we were young, and, we "crave" those tastes as adults, but refined, simple carbs have lost some things in the process of...processing. Vitamins for one, along with all the other nutrients that were present in the original whole food. The other thing taken out by refining...fiber. Less fiber means trouble, as we will see later in this book. So the message is: enjoy simple carbs as treats, but limit your intake. Fuel your body with a largely complex carbohydrate diet.

Chapter 10

Cholesterol and Fat (Triglycerides)

Keep in mind the Kiso Diet™ is not a low fat diet, but it is lower in fat than most diets. As you will see, not all fats are created equal. Let's first talk about Biomarkers...

Biomarkers...

Certain substances are found in the blood that coincide with diseases. For example, the presence of an antibody may indicate infection. These substances are known as biomarkers.

When looking at diet and disease, factors such as animal protein consumption relate directly to disease incidence, leading to changes in the concentrations of certain substances found in our blood. Those substances become biomarkers for disease. For example: **Blood cholesterol is a biomarker** for heart disease. Actually, the strongest predictor of disease *IS* cholesterol.

Did you know that we don't need to eat ANY cholesterol to be healthy? Our bodies have the ability to produce cholesterol if we don't supply it through our diets. And did you know that cholesterol in food comes **only** from animal sources? There is no cholesterol in a vegan diet!

In China, the average person's cholesterol is 127mg/dl compared with the average American's 215 mg/dl. There are those in America who actually say that having a blood cholesterol level of 150 mg/dl is too low and harmful for your health, but up goes cholesterol, and up goes heart disease. Did you know that when Dr. Campbell gathered information for his nutritional study, 85% of all Chinese had a blood cholesterol level lower than 150 mg/dl? And the death rate among Americans from diet related illness is 17 times higher than the Chinese! Excuse me, I'll take what the Chinese were eating please!

Americans are eating 33 to 40 percent of their daily total caloric intake in fat! The more animal products are eaten by a population, the more fat is consumed. Simple as that! Listen, lower fat means lower breast cancer rates too. So hear this...I said earlier that Americans eat over 20 plus percent of their diet in protein, but they also eat 33 to 40 percent of their diet in FAT! Holy C _ _ _ , or more accurately, Holy Cow!

When you have high cholesterol, you will more than likely have HIGH BLOOD PRESSURE. It's estimated that over 50 million Americans have high blood pressure. It's estimated that over one billion people the world over also have high blood pressure. As we have mentioned earlier in this book **thick blood causes atherosclerosis.** *The process is related to cholesterol.* Remember, there are two types of cholesterol in our bodies. There is the "good" cholesterol and the "bad" cholesterol. The good cholesterol is called HDL or *high density lipoprotein* and the bad one is called LDL or *low density lipoprotein.*

Your cholesterol and the level of your HDLs compared with your LDLs are biomarkers. Let's see how LDLs and high cholesterol aka "thick blood" work in your body.

In your arteries plaque, gathers around the bends and turns, (around your heart for example). Plaque is a kind of hard substance that occurs when the artery "scars" or when an artery needs repair.

Let's say your artery has some plaque. How did it get there? Most of it actually gets there through a process of repair. When the body gets a signals that there is a "leak" in the system, the body wages a tiny war. Platelets aggregate and stop the leak. The bad cholesterol, the LDLs, come to the rescue and act like a "foam" that is deposited over the repaired site causing the artery lumen (the inside of the artery) to become smaller. This causes less blood flow through the artery. This "bad" cholesterol, along with thickened blood causes this type of reaction not only around the heart but in all areas of the body.

Arteries have an ability to expand and contract. That's why when you get out of a hot tub, you feel light headed. This has occurred because the arteries in your body have responded to the heat and have dilated (or have become larger), allowing the blood to spread out, leaving less blood for your brain and causing you to feel "dizzy". It's worse if you're blonde...just kidding. This makes your blood pressure go down so when you suddenly stand, you feel faint. On the other hand, when you are freezing in the snow, your body's blood vessels constrict, making the blood slow down and causing a rise in blood pressure.

Well, as the process of the bad cholesterol takes place year after year, it causes the blood vessels to lose their ability to dilate and constrict. This is called hardening of the arteries or atherosclerosis, which I mentioned earlier. This is one of the processes that close down the small blood vessels in your brain which contributes to Alzheimer's disease. It eventually can cause your brain to not be as sharp as it was. It is also what's responsible for joint problems and sexual dysfunction and prostate problems in men, not to mention **heart attack** for god's sake.

Now, cholesterol is not all bad in that HDLs help "clean-up" or scavenge cholesterol from the body and carry LDLs back to the liver to be discarded. So if your HDLs are high and your LDLs are low, it's a better combo than having total low cholesterol but having your HDLs low and your LDLs high.

HDLs even help clean cholesterol from the artery wall where plaque has formed and can actually reverse atherosclerosis.

Individual cholesterol goals will vary depending on our own health situations, but here's a general guideline.

TOTAL: 200 or less

LDL: Less than 100

HDL: Higher than 60

The total count is significant, as is the ratio of LDL to HDL. Your LDL will usually be higher than your HDL, but the goal is for LDL to not exceed 3/4s of the total count, or a ratio of no greater than 3 to 1. Example: if your total is 200, LDL should be less than 150, which means HDL will be 50 or more. If you're advised you have high cholesterol and you're monitoring your levels, here's an easy way to remember it: you want to keep your overall count low, with your HDLs higher (remember H for HIGHER), and your LDLs lower (L for LOWER).

On to fats...

Not all fats are created equal! *Saturated or unsaturated...that is the question.* Well not exactly, but let's first look at **trans fatty acids**...really bad stuff!

The bad fats make your biomarkers for cholesterol much worse. These bad, bad fats are called trans fatty acids...the stuff in French fries and potato chips. This stuff is like genetically engineered material, it's not found in nature. It has been created in laboratories to enhance the ability of oil to withstand prolonged heating. It holds up very well when heated for long periods of time. Not surprisingly, trans fatty acids have an unnatural ability to last longer than "natural" oil. Perfect to stew in a McDonalds or a Wendy's for hours on end.

The process works like this...vegetable oil is heated with hydrogen gas. It causes a deadly mixture to form, called hydrogenated trans fatty acid or simply, hydrogenated or partially hydrogenated vegetable oil. It's found in baked goods and pastries, margarines, and all kinds of processed foods, so you have to read the labels of the food you are about to eat.

Recently, it's become a law that foods containing hydrogenated vegetable oils or trans fatty acids have to put it on the label for packaging. Very nice. Look at this statistic. "For every extra 2 percent of calories from trans fat daily— about the amount in a medium order of fast-food French fries—the risk of coronary heart disease increases by 23 percent. Eliminating trans fats from the U.S. food supply could prevent between 6 and 19 percent of heart attacks and related deaths" in the United States[2].

Also, the impact of trans fats on cholesterol are much worse compared with saturated fats. They raise bad LDLs and lower HDLs. That's why trans fats are not allowed in the Kiso Diet™ at all!

Saturated fats are also very bad for the system but eating some is absolutely acceptable on the Kiso Diet™. Saturated fats come mostly from animal source meats. We don't need to eat saturated fats in our diet at all because our body makes saturated fats if we need them. But getting a bit of your calories in the form of saturated fats cannot be avoided if you are a meat eater. Fish, chicken or fowl (always get it lean with the fat trimmed) are much lower in saturated fats compared with red meats like beef and pork, again your basic "mammalian" meats.

Also high in saturated fats are milk, cheese, sour cream, yogurt, and eggs. The problem with saturated fat from animal sources is that it will boost total cholesterol by elevating harmful LDLs. (remember, this increase in LDLs can make your blood thick). That's why in the Kiso Diet™, dairy, while

---

[2] From John Robbins' book ***The Food Revolution***.

not excluded, is not taken into the body in huge amounts, and milk is really avoided.

There are a few non-animal foods that contain saturated fats, like avocados, coconut milk, coconut oil and palm oil. Yes, these are saturated fats, but they are of a different chemical nature than animal-based saturated fats, and are digested easily. Once digested in the intestine, they are immediately taken to the liver for processing without any harm to the body. They also increase the metabolism, so they are seen in the Kiso Diet™ as acceptable saturated fats.

Unsaturated fats are considered "good" fats. They are predominantly found in foods from plants, such as vegetable oils, nuts, and seeds. However, there are two types of unsaturated fats, mono-unsaturated and poly-unsaturated.

Mono-unsaturated fats are found in canola oil, olive oil and avocados; and nuts such as peanuts, almonds, hazelnuts, and pecans; not to mention pumpkins and pumpkin seeds. Eating this kind of unsaturated fat is very good and actually raises the good HDLs and lowers the bad LDLs.

Poly-unsaturated fats are found in high concentrations in sunflower, corn, soybean, and flaxseed oils, and also in foods such as walnuts, flax seeds, and fish. *Now pay attention*, these fats have something very unique and good about them.

Remember I said that you don't "need" to eat saturated fats because you can make these in your own body when you need them? Well, there are some fats your body cannot make. We call these **Essential Fatty Acids** or **EFAs.** These fats you **must eat** in order to have them working in your body, and work they do. There are three types of EFAs. There are the **Omega 3s**, the "best," the **Omega 6s** and then the **Omega 9s.** Omega 3s are found in fish and fish oils, and good plant sources of Omega 3s are flax seeds and soy products. We will talk more about the Omegas later in the book.

One study found that replacing a carbohydrate-rich diet with one rich in unsaturated fat, **lowers blood pressure**, improves lipid levels, and reduces the estimated cardiovascular risk.

All these different types of fat mentioned above are **triglycerides.** *Triglycerides are also measured in your blood and used as biomarkers.* In general, the higher your triglycerides are, the higher your cholesterol and the higher your bad LDLs are.

The moral of the story is not to eat "low fat" but to eat the "right fat". So completely avoid hydrogenated trans fats and embrace vegetable sources of fats like olive oil and avocados. Significantly lower your intake of saturated fats by avoiding red mammalian meats and dairy products.

Chapter 11

The Glycemic Index

And the switch that shuts off your fat burning ability...

When you eat a meal, or anything for that matter, the presence of glucose, proteins in the form of amino acids, and fatty acids in the intestine, stimulate the pancreas to secrete a hormone called *insulin*. Insulin mostly acts on the cells of the liver, muscle and fat tissues of the body.

Insulin help the body absorb glucose, fatty acids and amino acids. It triggers the body to do two things: To stop releasing fat stored in your fat cells, and it stops the body from using fat present in the blood.

Insulin is regulated by an activity of lipoprotein lipases. If insulin is high, then the lipases are highly active; if insulin is low, the lipases are inactive. When the body does not have much insulin, the body is free to continue to release fat from fat stores when needed. In our human bodies, fat is continuously being released from our fat stores, and new fat is continuously being stored, depending on whether we need more fuel or we need to store fuel. After all, fat is stored primarily for fuel.

We have two types of fat cells. We have white fat cells and brown fat cells. White fat cells are designed to store energy for use in times of need. They are large cells; each one houses one large drop of fat. These big cells accumulate under the skin and around internal organs. They're the ones that accumulate in and around problem areas like the thighs on women and the stomach on men.

When you eat sugary stuff, it causes an insulin spike. This insulin spike causes the body to transform fatty acids found in the blood into fat molecules, and then to store them as fat droplets in white fat cells around the body. That's not good.

When insulin spikes, it is also possible for fat cells to take up glucose and amino acids which have been absorbed into the bloodstream after a meal, and convert them into fat molecules. This conversion of carbohydrates or protein into fat is 10 times less efficient than simply storing fat in a fat cell, but the body can do it. If you have 100 extra calories in fat (about 11 grams) in your bloodstream, fat cells can store it using only 2.5 calories of energy. Now look at this, if you have 100 extra calories in glucose (about 25 grams) circulating in your bloodstream, it takes 23 calories of energy to convert the glucose into fat and then store it. So it's much more efficient for the body to store fat in fat cells rather than taking the carbohydrates and proteins and storing them as fat. But the point is, the body can and does store carbohydrates and proteins as fat too. That's why it's wise not to over eat even good foods.

Now, let's look at insulin and different foods and why some cause that "insulin spike" and other foods don't. Our intestinal tract is about 20 feet long. When we eat complex carbohydrates (polysaccharide; starches & fibers) food travels through the entire gastrointestinal tract before it is processed completely. On the other hand, if you eat simple sugars (monosaccharides & disaccharides) they will be absorbed in the first foot of the small intestine. So, simple sugars (e.g. white bread, sugar) will be absorbed quickly in the small intestine, whereas whole grains (complex carbohydrates) will take about 20 feet to be absorbed. Because of this fact, simple sugars and simple carbohydrates will cause a rapid increase in blood insulin levels.

Now remember, if you cause your body to have lots of insulin in your blood because of what you have eaten, it will lower fat utilization because insulin will prevent the oxidation of fatty acids by blocking fats from entering the mitochondria. Therefore, insulin has the direct ability to prevent you from using fat for fuel.

What does this mean? It means you won't be getting rid of any fat for a while, until your blood insulin levels are naturally reduced, and this takes time. Generally, an insulin spike will take about 30 minutes to hit full force and about another 30 minutes to one hour to taper off. So if you are trying to lose weight, and you decide to have a glazed donut, BAM, your insulin is going to spike for about one hour or more. So for this amount of time you won't be reducing your fat stores. You also won't be burning any fat in your blood for that matter!

Now let's look at carbohydrates and how they impact the glycemic index.

Carbohydrates can be very sweet or not so sweet. All carbs have a glycemic index number. The sweeter the carb, the higher the glycemic number, and the less your body has to break it down to use it.

It may seem like a good thing to eat or drink something that the body does not have to break down because it's less work for your digestive system, but the opposite is true. The longer it takes your body to break down a carb, the more slowly its nutrients will arrive in your blood stream, impacting your insulin level. We call this impact "the hit."

If you eat honey your "hit" can be very quick, the glycemic index for honey is quite high. What this means is that when you eat a food that has a very high glycemic index, the faster it goes into your blood stream, the more insulin is called upon to get that sugar into your body for use. The more insulin that is called out to play, the faster you can get diseases like diabetes. In fact, this is what happens in type II diabetes. Your body has called two much insulin out too many times and the cells of the pancreas get tired and can't keep up with the demand and basically shut down. Excess sugar in your blood stream increases acidity in your body, which the body has to buffer. It does this by using calcium robbed from your bones to de-acidify your blood. And as we just discussed, the other bad thing about having an excess of insulin is that insulin tends to make the body store more, and burn less, fat!

So you see, that's why it's not great to eat lots of sugar, honey, or other highly sweet foods. It will call lots of insulin from your pancreas in order to use the sugar, then store that sugar as glucose inside your muscle tissue.

Since we are approaching the Kiso Diet™ as a cultural diet, we don't want to count all the numbers in the glycemic index. Just familiarize yourself with the glycemic index so you will have a working knowledge of which carbs cause a rise in acidity and insulin and which carbs don't.

You will notice by looking at the glycemic index that any kind of processed cereal is quite high compared with white rice (shredded wheat, for example, has a number of 69 compared to rice's 58). Take a look at this chart and see what things you like to eat and what number they have. The higher the number, the quicker the "hit." The quicker the hit, the more insulin is called out into the blood stream.

Remember this: The higher the glycemic index of a food, the more your body is "forced" to burn this carbohydrate because of the amount of insulin that comes out into your blood stream in response. With foods low on the glycemic index, less insulin is directed into the blood stream. Your body has the ability to burn fat and carbohydrates, but with lots of insulin floating in the system, your body shifts from burning fat to burning only carbs.

There is another important reaction that an insulin spike causes and that's a reduction in your natural production of Human Growth Hormone (HGH). The more insulin you have in your body, the lower the amount of HGH that is released from your pituitary gland. HGH is one of the most important hormones in your body and is directly related to muscle mass and fat retention. It's also directly related to aging. As we get older, less and less HGH is released making it harder for you to gain muscle and shed fat. There are natural ways to increase HGH, visit our website at kisodiet.com for more on hormone enhancement.

Food List	Rating Food Glycemic Index
Bakery Products	
Danish pastry	Medium, 59
Muffin	Medium, 62
Cake, tart	Medium, 65
Cake, angel	Medium, 67

Croissant ....Medium, 67
Waffles ....High, 76
Doughnut ....High, 76
Beverages
Soymilk ....Low, 30
Apple juice.....................................Low, 41
Carrot juice ....Low, 45
Pineapple juice.............................Low, 46
Grapefruit juice............................Low, 48
Orange juice...................................Low, 52
Breads
Multi grain bread......................Low, 48
Whole grain ....Low, 50
Pita bread, white.......................Medium, 57
Pizza, cheese ....Medium, 60
Hamburger bun ....Medium, 61
Rye-flour bread...........................Medium, 64
Whole meal bread ....Medium, 69
White bread................................High, 71
White rolls...................................High, 73
Baguette ....High, 95
Breakfast Cereals
All-Bran...Low, 42
Porridge, non-instant ....Low, 49
Oat bran ....Medium, 55
Muesli ....Medium, 56
Shredded Wheat ....Medium, 69

Golden Grahams......................High, 71
Puffed wheat...........................High, 74
Rice Krispies...........................High, 82
Cornflakes..............................High, 83

Grains

Pearl barley ....Low, 25
Rye...Low, 34
Wheat kernels ....Low, 41
Rice, instant ....Low, 46
Barley, cracked ....Low, 50
Rice, brown.............................Medium, 55
Rice, wild................................Medium, 57
Rice, white..............................Medium, 58
Barley, flakes..........................Medium, 66
Millet ....High, 71

Dairy Foods

Yogurt low- fat ....Low, 14
Milk, chocolate ....Low, 24
Milk, whole.............................Low, 27
Milk, Fat-free..........................Low, 32
Ice-cream ....Medium, 61
Ice-cream (low- fat)...............Low, 50

Fruits

Cherries ....Low, 22
Grapefruit...............................Low, 25
Apricots (dried)......................Low, 31
Apples....................................Low, 38

Pears................................Low, 38
Plums ....Low, 39
Peaches ....Low, 42
Oranges...........................Low, 44
Grapes.............................Low, 46
Kiwi fruit ....Low, 53
Bananas ....Low, 54
Mangoes ....Medium, 56
Apricots ....Medium, 57
Apricots (tinned in syrup) .Medium, 64
Raisins............................Medium, 64
Pineapple ....Medium, 66
Watermelon......................High, 72

Pasta

Fettuccine ....Low, 32
Vermicelli.........................Low, 35
Spaghetti, whole wheat......Low, 37
Spaghetti, white.................Low, 41
Macaroni ....Low, 45
Spaghetti, durum wheat......Medium, 55
Macaroni cheese................Medium, 64
Ravioli, meat filled ....Low, 39
Rice pasta, brown ....High, 92

Root Crop

Carrots, cooked.................Low, 39
Yam ....Low, 51
Sweet potato ....Low, 54

Potato, boiled.............................Medium, 56

Potato, new ....Medium, 57

Potato, tinned ....Medium, 61

Beetroot......................................Medium, 64

Potato, steamed ....Medium, 65

Potato, mashed ....Medium, 70

Chips...High,75

Potato, micro waved ....High, 82

Potato, instant...........................High, 83

Potato, baked ....High, 85

Parsnips..High, 97

Snack Food and Sweets

Peanuts ....Low, 15

M&Ms (peanut).........................Low, 32

Snickers bar................................Low, 40

Chocolate bar ....30g   Low, 49

Jams and marmalades..........Low, 49

Popcorn ....Medium, 55

Mars bar ....Medium, 64

Table sugar (sucrose)...........Medium, 65

Corn chips....................................High, 74

Jelly beans ....High, 80

Pretzels ....High, 81

Dates...High, 103

Soups

Tomato soup, tinned.............Low, 38

Lentil soup, tinned ....Low, 44

Black bean soup, tinned ......Medium, 64

Green pea soup, tinned........Medium, 66

Vegetables and Beans

Artichoke ....Low, 15

Asparagus...................................Low, 15

Broccoli......................................Low, 15

Cauliflower.................................Low, 15

Celery...Low, 15

Cucumber ....Low, 15

Eggplant.....................................Low, 15

Green beans...............................Low, 15

Lettuce, all varieties ....Low, 15

Peppers, all varieties.............Low, 15

Snow peas..................................Low, 15

Spinach......................................Low, 15

Young summer squash ....Low, 15

Tomatoes ....Low, 15

Zucchini ....Low, 15

Soya beans, boiled..................Low, 16

Peas, dried.................................Low, 22

Kidney beans, boiled.............Low, 29

Lentils green, boiled.............Low, 29

Chickpeas, dried ....Low, 33

Chickpeas, tinned ....Low, 42

Baked beans, tinned.............Low, 48

Kidney beans, tinned ....Low, 52

Lentils green, tinned.............Low, 52

Sweeteners

Agave Syrup.................................Low, 11

Brown Rice Syrup...................Low, 25

Maple Syrup ....Low, 54

Turbinado Sugar ....Medium, 65

White Sugar ....High, 80

High Fructose Corn Syrup..High, 87

Stevia, Stevita ....Low, 1

Honey..Medium, 55

I must warn you, I've seen people following the Kiso Diet do everything except reduce their sugar intake because of a sweet tooth. In reviewing their blood work, even though everything was better, they still had higher than should be triglyceride levels and higher LDLs which indicates that eating sugar laden foods or putting lots of sugar in your coffee can muck up the process! Try using agave for a sweetener. It does not cause the insulin spike that sugar causes. Even better yet, try Stevia for a sweetener, it does not cause an insulin rise at all. I like to use both agave and Stevita (Stevia) for a winning combo!

Chapter 12

The Three Forms of the Kiso Diet™

Vegan, Vegetarian, or Flexitarian?

Vegetarianism... The best diets by far for health are plant-based diets.

Plant-based diets are basically vegetarian diets. It is a known fact that when you are a true vegetarian, you live longer. If you eat right, you will decrease your total caloric intake compared with a meat eating diet. This alone can benefit, and therefore extend, your life. It is naturally a reduced calorie diet. You are healthier.

With a vegetarian diet you eliminate your propensity for a huge percent of all of the world's diseases. A lacto-ovo vegetarian diet gets rid of 40% of the world's diseases. If you are a vegan, meaning a vegetarian not eating any animal products at all (including dairy and eggs), you can get rid of up to 70 percent of the world's known diseases. (While healthier, being a vegan requires more expertise in knowing what to eat to get enough protein and nutrients, though our need for protein is much less than what most people think.)

More on Vegetarianism...

Many say that we are meant to be vegetarians. This could be true, considering most of the world's animals that have grasping hands are vegetarian. Consider our other physical attributes. Carnivores have claws...I cannot grow my nails more than 1/8 of an inch no matter what I do! Not that I'm trying... Look at human teeth. We don't have the sharp, serrated teeth or fangs which are found in the mouths of carnivores such as lions, tigers, and dogs etc. Our teeth provide flat surfaces for grinding, crushing and mashing plant matter, very much like the teeth of cows, elephants and other grazing herbivores.

Our intestines are 5 times longer on average than our own body length! Thus, we are suited for digesting plant matter since doing so requires a much longer time because of the indigestible cellulose and other tough fibers that are found in plant matter. Those same lengthy intestines create the perfect breeding ground for putrification of meat products in the intestine. Carnivores have a short intestinal tract which is well suited for the digestion of meat. Rapid eating, like a dog, and rapid elimination. No time for putrification. But the most compelling evidence is found in the fact that the more red meat you eat, the more heart disease you will have in general!

There is a great book written by Harvey Diamond called *Fit for Life*. I highly recommend it as the concepts are very good, though it may not be for everybody. He points out that most digestive problems come about by improper food combinations, and shows you how to eat the right combinations that can literally change your life.

Is a vegetarian lifestyle the only way to eat well? No. For many who enjoy meat, a vegetarian diet is just not tantalizing enough. That's why the Kiso Diet™ offers three choices. But what I've discovered by reading many books and by my own experience on a vegetarian diet is that we actually get enough protein from eating vegetarian. Over 50% of all vegans get more protein than their body can use, according to the China Study. I know it sounds odd from what we've been told, but it's true. Also, the more heavy protein you eat, the less calcium your bones absorb. Have you noticed that the animals with the largest bones on our planet are all vegetarian? Vegetarian diets have the most of something you need in your everyday diet and that's fiber.

Fiber

Fiber is an important consideration when it comes to any diet. **Did you know that fiber comes only from vegetable sources?** That's right, animal proteins and animal foods do not have fiber in them.

Fiber does many things! It pulls water from the intestines and gathers up toxic waste. Dietary fiber makes a person feel full. Eating fiber reduces the caloric density in our food. High amounts of dietary fiber decrease bowel and colon cancer. In China, where incidence of colorectal cancer (and diet related disease in general) is much lower than in America, dietary fiber intake is three times higher. The Chinese eat more veggies!

We will see later how to increase your fiber intake by cooking with the left over mulch of your juicer!

Let's imagine the food you eat passing through your digestive system, making its way to the other end. Your body absorbs nutrients, proteins, carbohydrates, and fats as the food passes through. Fiber eaten throughout the day assists the food on its journey. It adds bulk, allowing you to go to the bathroom everyday much more easily, and it acts like a broom, sweeping your colon over and over again. Plus fiber is a sponge, sucking up toxins and harmful waste products found in your intestines and colon, escorting them to their final exit.

Not only does fiber binds to toxins, fiber absorbs saturated fats from your digestive system, lowering the amount of cholesterol getting into your system. This is why it has been shown that eating oatmeal daily can lower total cholesterol. **Fiber keeps you less toxic and more healthy**.

To get enough fiber, you can make fiber cakes with the pulp left over from juicing your carrots and apples. Fiber cakes are very tasty and you can make a variety of good tasting things using your pulp. Another good fiber source is psyllium husks, a supplement which you can find cheaply at the health food store. Personally, I don't ever take the recommended amount of fiber supplements because I am already eating a fairly high fiber diet, so instead of taking two tablespoons full of psyllium husk fiber, I take only one. There is a disease state in Ayurvedic medicine, the six thousand year old healing system from India; a stickiness of your fecal matter called Ama. This Ama is one of the primary reasons for ill health in the Ayrurveda system of health. Eating lots of fiber will immediately make your stools less sticky and make going to the bathroom ten times easier!

When you are eating fibrous foods, be careful if you have conditions like diverticulitis or irritable bowel syndrome. These conditions can become active if you eat small seeds that can get caught in the folds of the intestine, making small infections happen and eventually leading to infection and pain. Small seeds found in strawberries or other berries for example can be bad for this. But for the average person, eating berries is just fine and add to a fiber rich diet.

Flexitarian Diet...

In the Kiso Diet™, you have the option to eat a flexitarian diet. What's a flexitarian diet? A diet where you eat as a vegetarian most of the time, and eat meat sparingly or once in awhile. It's been purported recently to be the "healthiest diet on the face of the planet" by some.

Why do many say these things?

A flexitarian diet gives you carbs plus allows you to eat some meats, giving you not only more repertoire and variety, but giving you "whole" proteins for added muscle building or body repairing qualities. Your fat intake is low, but you still enjoy the rich omega 3s from fish and fowl. Plus you get the health benefits of eating more veggies, more fruits and more grains. But probably most important, the Kiso Diet™ isn't a diet you go "on" or fall "off" of. It's a healthy way of eating that will suit you for life. That's why!

So, Vegan, Vegetarian or Flexitarian?

We need protein, as stated in Chapter 4 above. Animal proteins can promote cancer. One of the proteins that promotes cancer is casein protein, proved by information found in the China Study, the longest running nutritional experiment in the history of the world.

Does that mean you can't have any animal protein? No, it means not to have too much animal protein. Animal protein is a whole protein, meaning it has all the essential amino acids. In moderation, managed properly, this can be beneficial.

Exercise, Protein and the Kiso Diet™

Protein for body builders...

Exercise is part of the Kiso Diet™, right from the beginning. The Kiso Diet™ takes into consideration the needs of the athlete and the benefits of some consumption of animal protein. The basic Kiso Diet™, as laid out at the beginning of this book has three forms. A vegan form, a vegetarian form and a modified pesco vegetarian form (or flexitarian) form, allowing some meat and fowl.

Most people believe meat protein is necessary for strength and stamina. Before we get into more on which is better for athletes, eating meat or being vegetarian, let's look at an article found at the Food & Health web site: www.chineseop.com.

At Yale, Professor Irving Fisher designed a series of tests to compare the stamina and strength of meat-eaters against that of vegetarians. He selected men from three groups: meat-eating athletes, vegetarian athletes, and vegetarian sedentary subjects. Fisher reported the results of his study in the Yale Medical Journal. His findings do not seem to lend a great deal of credibility to the popular prejudices that hold meat to be a builder of strength.

"Of the three groups compared, the...flesh-eaters showed far less endurance than the abstainers (vegetarians), even when the latter were leading a sedentary life."

Overall, the average performance scores of the vegetarians were over double the average score of the meat-eaters, even though half of the vegetarians were sedentary people, while all of the meat-eaters tested were athletes. After analyzing all the factors that might have been involved in the results, Fisher concluded that: "...the difference in endurance between the flesh-eaters and the abstainers (was due) entirely to the difference in their diet.... There is strong evidence that a...non-flesh...diet is conducive to endurance."

A comparable study was done by Dr. J. Ioteyko of the Academie de Medicine of Paris. Dr. Ioteyko compared the endurance of vegetarian and meat-eaters from all walks of life in a variety of tests. The vegetarians averaged two to three times more stamina than the meat-eaters.

It's a known fact that vegetarians have more endurance than non vegetarians. It's also a known fact that vegetarian males have much less impotence and erectile dysfunction than meat eating males. Stamina isn't just a consideration for athletes! The problem of "erectile dysfunction" affects older (and sometimes not so old) males. What causes this? We're back to the hydraulic pump conversation! The blood vessels and veins that allow the penis to function are very small and are affected by the quality of the blood that runs through this area. When a person eats animal protein to excess, blood viscosity thickens, eventually causing erectile dysfunction to present itself.

It is said that vegans and vegetarians have a much longer shelf life when it comes to the bedroom department than the heavy barbeque crowd! Even on the flexitarian Kiso Diet™, you won't have the ill effects of "regular" meat eaters in this department, because you are balancing your meat eating with exercise. You're not eating mammalian red meats where the real saturated fats reside. The meat you are allowed to eat in the Kiso Diet™ has both omega 3s and a lower saturated fat content compared with mammalian red meats. Also you are exercising which helps lower the bad cholesterol and elevates the good cholesterol.

Need for protein...

In the Kiso Diet™, exercise is part of the deal. EVERYONE should exercise 30 minutes a day (you may combine two workouts and exercise for one hour, 3 times a week). If you are working out heavily, doing weight training, aerobics or running, etc., you can handle more protein than another person on the Kiso Diet™ who is not using his or her muscles as heavily.

When you exercise heavily, you've earned the right to eat more protein because your body uses more protein for muscle repair. A person who works out hard an extra 20 to 30 minutes a day will need up to 5% more protein in their diet. When you are doing the Kiso Diet™, you may, as an athlete, eat MORE protein (animal or plant-based) than the sedentary individual.

Remember I said that when a person consumed more than that golden percentage of 12% protein from their diet, cancer rates start to climb quickly? Well, if you are working out hard, you can increase this number by 5% without worry.

Here's the deal. After a protein consumption rate of around 12%, the cancer rate rises, so average exercisers should stay with 10%. If you work out hard, go ahead and eat 15%. As stated at the beginning of this book, you can eat fish, chicken, or turkey three times per week. This increase means you can have another piece of chicken, fish or turkey about the size of a playing card (20 grams of protein) for dinner on your workout days. If you are a bodybuilder or body sculptor, you may instead supplement with a protein shake on your workout days.

Any amount of animal protein that you eat OVER the amount your body NEEDS could promote cancer. So if you increase your need for protein by heavier exercise, you can safely eat more protein. Keep in mind that fish is a great protein source, but has possible pesticides and parasites, as mentioned earlier.

Isn't it funny that studies show that exercising with intensity can decrease cancer risk by 50%? Coupling this knowledge with the fact that exercising with intensity increases your need for protein by 50% is a perfect fit. Exercise more and you safeguard yourself from cancer and a whole host of other problems.

Chapter 13

What is a Whole Food, and more on Supplementation

One hundred years ago, 93% of our entire daily intake of food was from whole food sources. Today, only an estimated 7% of our daily intake of food comes from whole food choices for the average American. What happened?

Whole foods are not processed. Do you have to eat only whole foods on the Kiso Diet™? No. There is a diet from Japan called the macro-biotic diet where you eat mostly brown rice and other limited whole foods. Healthy, yes, but it gets pretty boring, I'm sorry. With the Kiso Diet™ not all the calories you eat have to come from whole foods. I think mixing things up with minimally processed foods like whole grain breads and other "health food" products (made from healthy ingredients) is the best overall way to eat. But one should strive to eat as much whole food as possible, at every meal. Eating fruits and vegetables with lots of potatoes (with skins) and brown (sweet) rice (it tastes good!), are key in Kiso Diet™.

Whole foods are so important! One school had suicides, violent confrontations, and drug and alcohol abuse during school hours among the students. Many students were carrying guns and weapons. In one year, this school changed from Pepsi machines, candy dispensers and processed junk foods on the menu to a plant-based, whole foods menu. Guess what happened? In one year there was not one violent crime, no weapons brought to school, no more violent altercations. There was also not one suicide after switching to a whole foods menu. Many of you may have heard about this. Now, many schools have followed suit and are also serving a plant-based whole foods menu!

Living on the Kiso Diet™, you should strive to have at least three whole foods with every meal. Best is a meal made of 100% whole foods like a salad, oatmeal, potatoes, etc.

What I mean by three whole foods at every meal is this: for dinner, you might have fish (a whole food), brown rice (a whole food) and tomatoes (a whole food). Simple as that, you've gotten your three whole foods! Then you can also have a minimally processed food (bread for example) with your meal. For lunch, you might have a burrito with lettuce, black beans and rice. Three whole foods with a tortilla (a minimally processed food). It all works together. And in combining beans with bread (or a tortilla), you create the perfect food, because while by themselves they both lack certain amino acids, taken together they make a whole protein!

When eating your diet from whole foods, you won't get any of the partially hydrogenated trans fatty acids mentioned earlier. That substance is not found in nature, so you won't find it in whole foods. What you will find is nature's synergy. We all know that mother earth has a great wisdom. Nature knows where to put things and what combinations work best for our bodies.

Sadly, our earthly environment has deteriorated over the past few hundred years from pesticide use and over farming. This has impacted the nutritional level of naturally grown foods all over the world. Some people feel they need to use supplements even though they are eating a whole foods diet.

Supplementation

The power of nature, in a pill or powder...

First let's look at medicines, and the pharmaceutical industry...Prescription medications, and even non-prescription supplements, are very big business. Very small chemicals synthesized from nature are being used to create powerful medicines, engineered to do very specific jobs, jobs the pharmaceutical companies want YOU to pay for. So much so that millions of advertising dollars are spent to motivate you to "ask your doctor" about medicines you've seen on television, promising to rid you of something dreadful you have, or to bring you something wonderful you're lacking!

The problem is, while these drugs may have been originally synthesized from nature, or at least, got their concepts from nature, their compounds are not found in nature at all. All the synergistic qualities found with herbs have been removed. What's left is a little tiny chemical or compound that causes a reaction in the body, a powerful reaction in the body. While this may relieve a particular symptom you have, it may cause other problems; the side effects we hear those commercials talking about... "So if you don't mind nose bleeds, temporary blindness and kidney failure, try our drug, because it will get rid of that redness around your nose!" Scary stuff. Most medications treat (or mask) symptoms. But few actually promote healing.

Year by year, people are becoming more savvy about medicines and their lack of healing power. It's driving more and more people like you and me towards a healthier life style, free from pharmaceuticals. Now, in this new millennia, people are taking control of their own health and not depending on the pharmaceutical industry to make them "healthy"!

Not that all drugs are bad, some will save your life! But the point is, eating your diet from whole foods as often as possible will give you nature's powerful synergy to sustain and keep your body in top shape. Your need for medications will be minimal.

On the Kiso Diet we juice. We may be juicing wheat grass or we may be juicing veggies or we may be using a blender to make smoothies and adding nutrients into the smoothie to enhance health. Some supplementation is good. **As we get older, there are some supplements in herb form that may help make the process of growing older easier. Find out more by visiting our website: www.kisodiet.com.**

Vitamins

If you don't like the taste of green drinks or don't have the time for juicing and find it easier to take a vitamin, try taking a very good whole food vitamin and mineral supplement. If they are separate, try taking the vitamin in the morning and the mineral supplement in the evening. Taking a vitamin that has basically all the essential nutrients once or twice a day is fine. It's also fine to take less than the recommended amount. If you find a whole food vitamin that recommends 8 pills a day but turns your urine green with just 4 pills, you are being over saturated! Try taking 2.

Taking a good whole foods vitamin that has an array of nutrients is better than taking many individual vitamins that have large amounts of one substance. For example, taking 4,000 times the RDA for Vitamin B1 would not be recommended! I personally like to make a smoothie in the morning, putting all my "stuff" in there. I open a capsule of my favorite whole foods vitamin and put the powder into my smoothie. I also add fun things like chocolate for flavoring. Healthy habits can be fun too!

Protein powders...

Protein powders are an easy way to add protein to your diet if you want more protein for building muscle, or for athletes in competition. Plus protein powders can add taste and texture to your smoothie, making it even more enjoyable. As said earlier, we easily get enough protein in our diets, so if you supplement with a protein powder, definitely use plant-sourced proteins like spirulina, hemp or soy.

Antioxidants

As I said earlier, we have potential cancer cells circulating in our bodies all the time. These potentially harmful molecules are highly reactive and can damage normal cells. That's where antioxidants come in. They intercept the potentially harmful reactive cells and neutralize them with an electron that makes them harmless.

See the fantastic color of different fruits and vegetables? The color tells us they're loaded with healthy antioxidants. The higher the vibrancy of color, the more antioxidants there are in those wonderful things. Eat at least 3 to 5 whole fruits per day. Bananas, apples, oranges, watermelon... eat all kinds of fruit!

I believe it's best to get antioxidants naturally through a healthy diet, but you can also take them in supplement form. If you feel you need more antioxidants, you can look into vitamin C, vitamin E, co-Q10, or resveritrol, the "new" antioxidant that has been touted as the "best" antioxidant you can take to help slow the aging process.

Aging is said to be "uncontrolled free radical damage." I believe this to be true. You make the choice and take antioxidants in supplement form if you like, but I prefer having nature on my side with all the synergistic vitamins and minerals in a natural antioxidant juice. You can get a huge amount of antioxidants from juicing or wheatgrass.

Anti-Inflammatories...

Some foods have natural anti-inflammatory properties. Onions are great! They are high in quercetin, a type of antioxidant that inhibits the enzymes that trigger inflammation; onions also contain sulfur compounds that are used to manage the body's immune system. Other good sources of quercetin include apples, broccoli, red wine, red grapes or grape juice and tea.

To supplement, you can take a good "joint health" remedy, made with the right combinations of anti-inflammatory agents like boswellia and turmeric (a list can be found on our website, kisodiet.com). And remember, stress and the function of your immune system play huge roles in inflammation, as does what you DON'T eat.

Junk foods, sugar and fast foods will increase inflammation in your body. This is partially due to the unhealthy fats used in preparing and processing these foods. Trans fatty acids and saturated fats are other things to avoid. Processed meats such as lunchmeats, hot dogs and sausages are high in fats and also contain chemicals such as nitrites that are associated with increased inflammation and chronic disease.

Avoid most dairy products if you are trying to reduce inflammation. You don't need the extra saturated fat. Saturated fats are also found in meats, dairy products and eggs. Additionally, these foods also contain fatty acids called arachidonic acid. While some arachidonic acid is essential for your health, too much arachidonic acid in the diet may make your inflammation worse. Chicken has lots of arachidonic acid. If you want to get rid of possible arachidonic acid in foods like chicken, you have to heat the foods up to over 180 degrees F.

Good food is the best medicine

"Supplements" are just that, supplements. Added extras. Unless you have unusual needs, with a healthy diet, you'll have minimal needs for additional antioxidants or complicated vitamins. The best practice is simply to eat well, juice, and look to nature for the beautiful, whole foods, ready to make you healthier!

Chapter 14

Getting Enough Nutrition and Not Getting the Bad Stuff…GMO Foods

Balanced diets and nutritious foods

The traditional **Japanese diet** is good because it is mostly a fish, rice and vegetable diet. Keep in mind, however, that raw fish can have parasites and can also be loaded with pesticides. Large fish eat other smaller fish, absorbing all their toxins and pesticides that may be found in their bodies. Cooking can eliminate some of these toxins, but not all. That's why, in the Kiso Diet™, we don't eat shellfish, they are bottom dwellers and harbor many bad agents, and I advise you to limit fish consumption to three times a week, maximum.

Also the Japanese traditionally eat vegetables, seaweeds and fruits that are in season. This is very good for homeostasis (maintaining internal stability). Eating cold foods in a cold climate (for example, eating a green salad with cucumbers in Siberia in winter) would not be recommended.

The **Mediterranean diet** also has cooked fish and lots of rice and veggies as well, which is very good for you and tasty at the same time.

Fruit

How about fruit? Many believe that, as human beings, our hands are designed to grasp fruit. Look at the shape of a banana or an apple. They are perfect for the human grasp. Also our teeth are very fruitarian in design. Eat a lot of fruit, especially when it's fresh and as organic as possible, but eat it on an empty stomach.

So many times we eat fruit after or during a meal, but this creates a sour stomach. Fruit digests very quickly, so if you eat fruit with a carbohydrate, it backs up the digestive process and makes the quickly digesting fruit sit in your intestines. It ferments and becomes putrid causing gas and bloating.

If you eat fruit first thing in the morning, or in the mid-afternoon when you haven't eaten for at least two hours prior, you will have no ill effects; in fact, fruit is 70% distilled water! This is great for your digestive tract and helps you eliminate well.   That's why if you eat fruit by itself, it passes right through the intestines delivering its antioxidant-rich nutritional value before passing through as waste.

Meat

If you love meat, eat it sparingly, combining it correctly so you don't develop an upset stomach. Also, try eating only chicken and different fowls. Steaks should be eaten only occasionally because even a lean steak is still about 60% fat! You take things in: water, salts, food, oils and must process them through your body. Imagine the grease found in one steak caught in a filter. Yes, your body has to filter that steak too and the grease sticks to things like your digestive tract and arteries! Just keep this in mind.

Juicing

Juicing, taking wheatgrass or taking a green drink daily will make you feel better and have more energy. Wheatgrass is fantastic! Remember to reduce your total caloric intake on a daily basis, which will help you feel that much better. You won't be taxing your body as much. Also taking a green natural drink or juicing instead of overloading yourself with vitamins will alleviate much of the workload on your kidneys and other organs to maintain homeostasis.

Have you ever heard of the "Juice Man"? He's Jay Kordich, the guy that used to advertise his Juiceman juicer a few years back. In 1948, at the age of 25, Jay was diagnosed with bladder cancer. A world-class athlete and football star at USC, Jay found Dr. Max Gerson, who helped Jay cure himself of bladder cancer using a vegan diet and juicing. From that time on, Jay started telling all he knew about the benefits of juicing. Jay is in his 80s now and looks and feels great. He personally likes to juice carrots and apples, among other things. By the way, you can still buy a Juice Man juicer at many outlets around the United States and online.

I recommend you either juice once a day with a vitamix-type juicer (which mixes the pulp with the juice for added fiber) or juice with a "regular" juicer that separates the pulp from the juice, and save the pulp to make healthy snacks. The other options are two: juice wheatgrass with a simple wheatgrass juicer, or if you cannot do the above then make a smoothie with a "green" drink powder, they are very good also. For more on juicing, visit us at: kisodiet.com.

White foods

One rule of thumb: cut down on white foods. Reducing or eliminating white foods like milk, sugar, creams, salt, white bread, and white flour is a good idea. Reducing these foods and substances tend to make the job of maintaining homeostasis easier.

Now for the really bad stuff... GMO products...

It all started with a Supreme Court ruling that made it legal for a person (or company) to patent life! In the 1980 landmark case of Diamond v Chakrabarty, the US Supreme Court ruled that a living organism, a bacterium that could digest oil, could be patented. Bioengineering for profit was born... Who did this benefit, you ask? Listen to this.

After the Supreme Court decision, corporate investors hugely benefited! A few months after the ruling, a recently formed biotech company called Genentech offered a million shares of stock to the market at $35 per share. After just 20 minutes, the shares were being sold at $89. By the end of the day, the company had raised $36 million. Genentech had not yet introduced a single product onto the market, yet made millions of dollars.

Bioengineered crops are now HUGE business. Most genetically engineered crops planted worldwide are designed either to survive exposure to certain herbicides, or to kill certain insects. The herbicide the plants are modified to survive is the active chemical agent "Round-up." Round-up is manufactured by a company called Monsanto Corporation. Guess who has the patent on life that we spoke of earlier? You guessed it, Monsanto Corporation! They modified plant genes to withstand their own product, Round-up. The other funny thing (not so funny!), is the deep ties of the Monsanto corporation to both the FDA and the USDA. In spite of objections over the blatant conflicts of interest, upper echelon executives of the Monsanto Corporation have been appointed to both the FDA and the USDA... showing how closely related Monsanto Corporation is to the government agencies responsible for monitoring its products and practices...Scary!

The United States is the largest producer of corn in the world. Corn is the largest crop grown in the United States, with soybeans a close second. Approximately 80% of all US corn and 90% of soybeans are GMO. Much of that is consumed by livestock, which we, in turn, ingest by consuming non-organic animal products. We also consume it in corn and/or soy oil, high fructose corn syrup, and a plethora of other processed food products. GMO is major, major, **big business**!

How about the harmful effects of GM foods...

Scientists in Russia have proven that GM foods are disastrous. In April of 2010, Russian scientists proved that animals fed GM foods had profound changes in their health and function. In the study, one group of hamster cubs was fed non-GM soya (hard to find in Siberia, where the study was done, as 95% of the soybeans grown there are genetically modified). A 2nd group of hamster cubs was fed genetically modified soya. After three generations, the cubs fed GM soya could no longer reproduce. GM foods were the sole cause.

Here's another interesting piece of information. All that GM corn that's being fed to livestock isn't doing the animals (or the people who eat their meat) any favors. Cows are built to eat grass, not corn. Cows raised on corn require huge quantities of antibiotics to keep them "healthy" and free of disease. Antibiotic residue remains in the animal meat, and is absorbed into the human body when we eat it, creating antibiotic resistance in humans. If you eat beef, and want to avoid GM corn and antibiotics, buy organic, grass-fed beef.

In a 1999 report, the British Medical Association, the leading association of doctors in Britain, urged an end to the use of antibiotic resistance genes in genetically engineered crops. "There should be a ban on the use of antibiotic resistance marker genes in GM [genetically modified] food, as the risk to human health from antibiotic resistance developing in micro-organisms is one of the major public health threats that will be faced in the 21st Century. The risk that antibiotic resistance may be passed on to bacteria affecting human beings, through marker genes in the food chain, is one that cannot at present be ruled out," the Association said.

We don't know enough about GM foods and in my opinion, we should not mess with genetically modifying anything! One of the biggest reasons for shopping at the health food store is to guard yourself against consuming GM foods!

In one recent study from Yale University found that rats, fed GMO soy in three generation could not have offspring anymore and grew HAIR inside their mouths…that's disgusting!

I'm telling you, you don't want to mess with nature. **GM foods can alter your DNA, change your brain waves, and can even destroy your immune system, your organs and can make you infertile.**

Chapter 15

Kiso Diet™, Body Typing and your Motivation to Change

Here's what happens when you eat the Kiso Diet™ way. The Kiso Diet™, as you know, has three phases. The reason for this is that not everyone is the same. Some folks make a choice to be vegetarian or vegan even though their bodies, or their minds for that matter, may not at first be suited to that diet.

For example: You have Tom, he is a pitta type body (more on body types later). Very athletic, big muscles, but he may be tired most of the time. (This happens when you eat lots of protein and saturated fats. It's due to the fuel. If your fuel is heavy, you will feel heavy.) As Tom changes his eating patterns, his body will start to generate energy by switching from his old diet of saturated fats and lots of meat, to a complex carb diet, with lots of grains and vegetables. Carbohydrates will make Tom's body burn faster because it's easier for a body to burn carbohydrates (remember, carbs are in the preferred gas tank). He'll feel better, but he's got some big adjustments to make, mentally and physically.

In the China Study, Dr. Campbell found that people eating a good "carbohydrate" diet tend to burn off their calories as heat coming from their bodies. I stated this earlier in this book. This, in itself, will cause weight or fat loss. It's a healthy way to burn fat. There are lots of other theories about diet out there to choose from, ranging from healthy to un-healthy. I would consider all of the "quick" weight loss diets to be unhealthy. Furthermore, I would say that the Atkins diet and the South Beach Diet are both unhealthy. In other words, I would deeply council my kids to reconsider if they were going to go on one of these diets, because I care for their health. But there are some healthy diets that are vastly different than the Kiso Diet™. Let's look at a few.

There is the macrobiotic diet from Japan. Dr.Kushi, the founder of the macrobiotic diet, had his followers eat whole foods, nothing processed. He also had folks eating brown rice almost at every meal. It's healthy, but few stay on this diet for very long...boring!

Harvey Diamond, in his book *Fit for Life*, talks about the benefits of a vegetarian diet compared with a diet allowing meat, and addresses proper food combining. I mention his book a few times in *The Kiso Diet*™ because I think he has some valid points. Many people follow his food combining tips throughout their lives due to the fact that it makes digestion easier.

Weston A. Price was a pioneer of nutrition and studied indigenous peoples around the world, when they were still following their natural native cultural diets. In his book **Nutrition and Physical Degeneration**, 1930, Price gives an example of how indigenous Eskimos and Indians of Alaska ate a high saturated fat diet coming from whale blubber and red meats, but had almost no heart disease or disease of any kind. But once these "natives" started living in towns and cities and started to adopt the white man's diet, their wonderful, lustful health quickly deteriorated into ill health. One interesting fact that Price found was that these indigenous cultures ate food that had approximately four times the nutritional value compared with our current foods grown in America. (This current loss of nutritional value is due to our land's loss of nutritious soil from over farming, and food production.)

From Price's studies, other nutritionists started writing their books, one of which was very pivotal called **The Metabolic Typing Diet**. The author, William Wolcott, put many concepts together. He took his cue from Watson and Kelley who, earlier on, noticed a relationship with the two parts of the autonomic nervous system (ANS), called the sympathetic and the parasympathetic nervous system. The sympathetic nervous system is often called the "fight or flight" part of your nervous system. He believed people who operate from this side of the ANS need certain foods, and people running on the parasympathetic side of the ANS need another set of nutrients. Their idea was that you could balance the two sides of the ANS through diet. This would restore balance within the individual and restore health. They also found that some individuals were "fast oxidizers," they burned their food quickly. The rate at which your cells convert food into energy determines whether you are a fast oxidizer or a slow oxidizer.

William Wolcott found that "the dominance factor" was the key to putting together a typing profile that many people found helpful in getting themselves back on the road to health. He put it all together in his book *The Metabolic Typing Diet*. One of the points he made in his book was that individuals have either a sympathetic dominance or a parasympathetic dominance.

He said that people are too different to have one diet work for everyone. He believed some needed high "purine" (acidic) saturated fats like red meats, pure milk, and cheese, in order to heal. Others needed a high complex carb diet low in fats and proteins. He would place his patients into a metabolic type and then prescribe a diet for that individual.

Even with Wolcott's profound knowledge about metabolic typing, many patients did not find health at all.

I agree with the value of body typing, but not in the same way as Wolcott's *Metabolic Typing Diet,* with the different typing categories based on sympathetic vs. parasympathetic nervous system types. In my clinic, we work with the parasympathetic and sympathetic nervous systems every day.

Yes, most folks have a dominant side, but this shouldn't be reinforced with diet. It can, and should, be changed!

Say we have Joan, who comes in with what we call sympathetic over-ride. Light hurts her eyes, she cannot sleep well. She is tired not from her para-sympathetic nervous system being "on" too much, but from her sympathetic nervous system being "on" too much. She has what we call adrenal burnout. She may also have anxiety and panic attacks with this condition because she is in a state of fight or flight. Do I want to give her a diet for her sympathetic override, or her constant state of fight or flight? No, I want to get her out of that state. Because in that state she will never be fully healthy, or happy for that matter.

Employing Kiso Method™, I can change Joan's sympathetic override by manipulating her upper neck and cranium in a very specific manner that will alleviate pressure on her cranio-sacral region and bring back the balance of her para-sympathetic nervous system. And through stress management and relaxation techniques, we can make her balanced again. If I were to give her a diet high in animal proteins and saturated fats, this would prolong and engrain her fight or flight constitution. But by going to the core of her sympathetic override and constant state of fight or flight, we can give her a diet that will calm her down to go along with "changing" her condition from agitation to rest and relaxation! A diet that is vegan or vegetarian may aid in her recovery.

Yes, I can see that we are all individuals and have different needs (based on body type, personality, tastes, philosophies, mindset...) but we are all people. I don't believe anyone needs high "purine" saturated fats and proteins in their diet on a regular basis just because their body type is different from another person's body type. I say the reason indigenous Eskimos tolerated red meat and whale blubber without getting heart disease was due to the fact that they ate tons of salmon! Already stated in this book was the outcome of an experiment where individuals on a diet of salmon dropped their triglyceride levels by 47%! That's huge! This is the power of ingesting omega 3s, and why, in the third phase of the Kiso Diet™, we have the option of eating fish. Omega 3s not only help repair atherosclerosis, but keep it from happening. Also omega 3s taken daily help inflammation in the body. Very positive stuff!

I readily accept that as individuals we have different needs. One reason I made the Kiso Diet™ with three different forms is for just this very reason. We are all different, mentally and physically, but not soooo different, if you get my drift. People are people.

While the Kiso Diet™ is designed to provide flexibility, the beginning of the Kiso Diet™ is the same for everyone. We start with a vegan diet for one week, then move to the lacto-ovo vegetarian form of the Kiso Diet™ on the second week. If you wish to eat meat or fish, you'll be practicing the flexitarian side of the Kiso Diet™, which you will begin on your third week.

When first embarking on the Kiso Diet™, you may possibly have some lag time for a few weeks. It will be a time of cleansing. If you've been running on saturated fats and proteins, like Tom at the beginning of this chapter, your body has to get used to running on complex carbs, a lower amount of protein, and a different type of fat (you've moved from saturated fats to monounsaturated and polyunsaturated fats). All good stuff, but you may notice changes in your body until you get used to running on this new fuel. The changes you feel may be varied. Again, if this were Tom, he might feel gassy (due to an increase of plant based foods) or he might feel slightly tired, but in a few weeks he should start to thrive!

So after the initial 3 weeks, do you go vegan, vegetarian, or flexitarian? It's up to YOU! You're the one to decide. I say it's your mind, not your body type, that determines whether or not you are a vegetarian or a flexitarian. Some on the Kiso Diet™ want to be pure vegans. No meat, no dairy, just pure vegetables. That's fine. They are mentally prepared for it. They "want" it. For whatever reasons, maybe health or spiritual, they are done with eating meat. If they have this mind set, I believe their bodies will shift to accept this new way of eating.

For some people being a vegan is too stringent perhaps, so they adopt the lacto-ovo vegetarian diet. These folks may opt for this because they like seasonings or dressings that contain dairy and want to have an egg once in awhile. Or maybe they want to be on the flexitarian diet because they love fish or chicken and don't want to exclude these things from their diet. On the flexitarian diet, if you want to work out six days a week to have the option of eating an animal protein every day (except one day a week), that's fine.

We are all individuals and as individuals we have the right to choose the diet that's best for ourselves. Following any part of the Kiso Diet™, whether it's the flexitarian, vegetarian or vegan, one thing is for sure, IT'S BETTER FOR THE ENVIRONMENT! Eating less animal protein, especially less mammalian animal protein helps our soil to regain its nutrients. Basically, according to John Robbins in his book **Diet for a New America**, we help feed the planet by eating more vegetarian. Maybe hardcore vegans will point a finger at me, but any phase of the Kiso Diet™ is not only healthy, it's good for the environment.

Body typing is as easy as 1, 2, 3!

I do believe there's truth in the concepts of body typing. But the Kiso Diet™ looks at body typing differently than the metabolic typing diet talked about above. In fact, The Kiso Diet™ is different than any diet out there right now in the world of diet books.

We use the three body types, or doshas, listed in Ayurveda. Ayurveda has a history of about six thousand years and is the main indigenous healing system of India. Ayurveda establishes we have three body types.

1. Type one, what we call a **vata type**, is a lean person, usually tall and more gangly, a fast oxidizer. This person usually can eat lots without gaining weight. This person likes to read and think a lot. This person is often nervous and has trouble relaxing.

2. Type two, what we call a **pitta type**, is usually muscular and athletic and can easily lose weight or gain weight depending on the circumstances. This person is usually athletic and can have a bad temper. This person likes to move but can rest when needed.

3. Type three, what we call a **kapha type**. This person is heavy and usually has a hard time losing weight. Even if they don't eat much, they find it difficult to lose weight. Their energy is usually slow and they have a tendency to lie around.

Each type can be a mixture of one or two of the other types. This mixture can be not only a physical trait, but a personality trait or a mental trait. For example, a pitta type may have vata characteristics but not have any characteristics of a kapha. You may have a pitta type body, muscular and athletic, but a vata mind, always thinking and worried all the time. (Of course there are wonderful things about a vata mind! I have one!) What ever your type is, you can balance it to blend in other doshas to make yourself healthier.

Exercise will help all the doshas. The pitta will burn some excess energy and work the muscles allowing that individual to thrive. Eating a flexitarian diet may be best for this person. But the determining factor is that person's mind. Does he or she want to change their dosha a bit, becoming more of a vata type person? This is up to the individual. The combination of one's wants and desires coupled with the trying out a new way of eating and seeing how it fits will be the answer. They may find that having a pitta dosha or being "hot tempered" is something they want to change. Food can help change this, also relaxing more and doing something more sedentary can help...like reading a book or watching the ocean. You might find a kapha type person dreaming to be an athletic type individual. Exercise and eating on the flexitarian diet is just the ticket for them. Or a Kapha type wanting to become a lean yogi type and the vegan diet will be suited for that.

In picking which form of the Kiso Diet™ is best for you, you'll want to take also look at your dosha for what it is. If you are a kapha and you have been over weight for most of your life and perhaps have high blood pressure and heart disease, you can go on any form of the Kiso Diet™ and find improved health, but which phase of the Kiso Diet™ you prefer will depend on which appeals most to you. You might decide the flexitarian diet is not what you want, and drop into a vegetarian diet or vice-versa. But I will tell you facts about the Kiso Diet™ that will make you healthier regardless of your body type.

The Kiso Diet™ is low in animal fat or has no animal fat. It's lower in saturated fats. It's a largely organic diet and accordingly has fewer preservatives and chemicals. The Kiso Diet™ is low in milk consumption and dairy products, which cuts your cancer rate. The diet is low in animal protein, which again lowers your cancer risk and lowers your intake of hormones and possible diseases from animals. Finally, the Kiso Diet™ has you exercising which not only lowers cancer risk again but battles atherosclerosis and turns your bad cholesterol to good cholesterol! All this will make you move into your proper weight, which will usually be vastly lighter than you are now. Being lighter and exercising more will bring more vitality to your daily life.

Now on to weight loss!

Chapter 16

Weight loss and the Kiso Diet™

Weight loss is a natural outcome while on the Kiso Diet™. As Dr. Campbell says in his book The China Study, people eating a plant-based complex carbohydrate naturally burn more calories than a person on the SAD diet. Even though they eat more (you will never starve on the Kiso Diet!), than people on the SAD diet, they burn their extra calories in the form of heat. I said "weight loss is a natural outcome while on the Kiso Diet." Let's rephrase that; weight loss is a natural occurrence while living your LIFE with the Kiso Diet™. You don't have to count calories anymore. Eating a plant-based, whole foods oriented diet, but still having the luxury of eating healthful snacks, flavoring with cheeses and even having an occasional steak if you want it will result in weight loss for 85% of the those following the diet! That's right. If you are very overweight, it's going to be AMAZING! DON'T count calories anymore for the rest of your life.

Knowing that eating refined sugars and carbohydrates causes insulin to soar is in itself useful knowledge. When insulin soars, you stop burning fat in your blood stream and you stop burning fat in your fat stores. That's why exercise works 300% better at burning fat when done in the morning! Your insulin levels are at their lowest. Practicing the Kiso

Diet™, eating mostly whole foods, will keep your insulin levels on the low side most of the time.

The Kiso way of eating gives your body suppleness with strength, all at the same time. How is this done? Having a low blood viscosity oxygenates all the cells of your body; including your heart, your brain and your joints, just to name a few areas. Because of this your body will have endurance and energy you have never thought possible before. Because YOU choose which diet is right for you in the Kiso Diet™, you can change your physical self from someone who is 35 pounds (or 100, for that matter) overweight and tired all the time, to someone you only thought possible in your dreams. A lithe, slender, supple, yoga practitioner; or a muscular but flexible athletic type; or the person you've always wanted to be!

With the Kiso Diet™, I recognize how dreams affect you. They motivate you! Dreams are how everything in existence was manifested! Everything you do in your life, everything you have in your life, was first "dreamed" by you, whether you know it or not! So dream away. Sure, if you are big boned and the yoga master type is your dream ideal, you will have your own version of that. But life is fun and exciting, don't let other people tell you what you can be, make yourself into *your* ideal type.

One time about 15 years ago while I was practicing in Monterey, California, I found a newspaper article. Here was a picture of an older man, a yoga teacher in the L.A. area. He was lithe, had a bald head and a long grey goatee. He was muscular but slender and the newspaper photos showed him teaching his class and doing some amazing yoga moves himself. The man pictured in the newspaper looked like a yoga master for sure to me. I was fascinated! Well, as I read the article, I was deeply touched by his personal story. At around 55 years old, he was homeless, an alcoholic and 50 pounds overweight. He suffered a heart attack and was rushed to the hospital. The doctor told him that he had been lucky *that* time and would make it but, if he did not change his lifestyle and change his ways, that he would surely die.

Well, this man took these words to heart and as the article said, "He became the most sought-after Yoga teacher in the L.A. area, and he was 72 years old!" Wow, that's changing things up! How many of his acquaintances at the time of his heart attack would have believed him if he had told his friends that he was going to change his life and lose 50 pounds and become the most sought after yoga teacher in L.A.? Nooooooo one! So, often times it's good to keep your dreams to yourself. Your friends and relatives will surely notice what you are doing and become curious, but don't listen to negative feedback from others. Many folks don't want to change themselves, or perhaps they don't believe they *can* change themselves. Don't let them project their negativity on you. Your dreams are your dreams and you deserve the pleasure of attaining those dreams!

The Yin and Yang of life and food...

The power of nature and the Universe is based upon yin and yang principals. That's why it is so important to balance your diet with yin and yang foods and yin and yang cooking.

Our body is basically made to work with the rhythms of nature. When we wake up in the morning, we are set for elimination (a bowel movement), then we want breakfast (or vice versa). Some say to eat your biggest meal in the morning, but it's a yang time in the Kiso Diet, so it's not good to load up your stomach because the morning is when we should expend the most energy of the day. Eat lightly (yin), but enough to sustain you until snack time. We have snacks once, between each meal. Eating fruit in the morning is great after exercise. Fruit is 70% distilled water, so it's easy to digest; eaten alone is best for digestion.

Lunchtime is between yin and yang. Eating a medium amount is good. If you eat a heavy, protein-laden lunch, serotonin will hit you after you eat and you will feel the need to sleep. That's why in Spain they have siesta time, so people can take a nap after eating lunch.

Nighttime (the beginning of the evening) is more yin and you need to eat more protein (yang) at dinner. Protein is hard to digest, but you will relax after dinner, so it's a better time to eat your protein.

Basically pressure cooking, or heavily cooking, makes any food yang, that's why pressure cooking is good for vegans. Because the vegan diet is very yin, you need the yang style of pressure cooking in order to, sometimes, balance this. Lightly cooking food, or not cooking at all, creates yin foods. Proteins and fats are more acidic in the blood and are considered yang in the Kiso Diet™. Complex carbs and vegetables are considered yin foods. Fruits are also considered yin because they are not cooked and full of water.

So those folks eating tons of steak for lunch and hamburgers for dinner and sausage and eggs for breakfast are piling the YANG on top of YANG which means they are getting more and more ACIDITY in their blood which creates URIC ACID and that's why people get GOUT! Too much yang. Couple this with alcohol, which by the way is a yang, and you get way too much yang in your system and your body can have all kinds of reactions like swollen joints and auto immune diseases. In the same vein, those on a raw food diet get way too much yin, but it's great for curing diseases that were originally caused by eating way too much yang, which is normally the case.

Also, I might mention something very important here. If you drink cold drinks at dinner...it's very bad. In Chinese medicine your stomach is the furnace. It's burning and processing your food. It's like an oven...you don't throw ice water in your oven! Cold drinks at any time are usually not good unless you're hot and have been physically working prior to consuming the cold drink. Warm or hot drinks are much better for the harmony of your body's yin and yang qualities!

If you are a vegan, you are on a yin diet. It's great for many people. Of course, it won't work for everybody. I've seen many people try but not be able to go for more than a few months without having to either become a lacto-ovo vegetarian or to start eating some kind of meat. Perhaps their body constitution is very yin to begin with and learning to eat as a vegan is not so easy.

That's why I mention at the beginning of this book that being a vegan for short periods of time in order to heal something like diabetes or joint inflammation or heart disease or cancer works tremendously well. But carrying this diet on for more than one year takes vigilance and expertise. As I have said previously, YOU can decide what YOU want to do.

If you find it wrong to eat animals and dairy products, if you truly decide being vegan is your new life style, go for it. See how you feel. A *metabolic body typing* practitioner may tell you that you can't be a vegan. I believe you can dream yourself into what your heart truly desires. If a vegan diet is the only diet you want in your life (whatever your reasons), then go for it! Just remember, eating vegan requires eating many different types of foods from fruits to root vegetables to plant-based protein-rich foods. Don't worry, we have all of these foods in Mother Nature's chest of drawers...it just takes some experimenting and knowledge to carry it out. You can do it if you truly desire it. I believe through the power of your mind, you can change your own body constitution!

Why do I say this? Because I've seen it done many, many times, by many individuals. What often has made a person's "body constitution" in the first place was not nature, it was nurture, mom's pot roasts and mom's apple pies! Eating this way for 18 years will cause a person to develop a certain body constitution. Looking at this individual from the outside, a metabolic typing practitioner would say "no, a vegan diet is not right for you." They may say you need an animal protein and high saturated fat diet because that's your constitution. I say it's your constitution *currently*, but I believe knowing about blood thickness, and the harms of eating diary products, and drinking milk, and how diets high in animal proteins are not good for anyone, will change your mind and send you searching for a new constitution!

The metabolic typing folks say that we are all "human," meaning we are highly individual and we require different fuels to satisfy these differences. In Wolcott's book **The Metabolic Typing Book**, he says that we require different fuels because we are so individualized as human beings. I say, yes we are different in our doshas, but we are similar in that we are basically designed the same.

Liken this to a gas burning car. If you burn diesel fuel in a car designed to burn regular gas, the engine will clog up fast, causing lots of problems in a short amount of time.

I believe this is what's happening with heart disease and diabetes and a whole host of other diseases stemming from high animal proteins and saturated fats. WE ARE SIMPLY NOT DESIGNED TO RUN ON THESE "HEAVIER" FUELS. This is precisely why dogs (canines) are able to eat meat, day in and day out and not have any heart disease...they were designed that way. Their teeth, stomachs, intestines and livers are of a carnivore design. We are obviously, as human beings, not of a carnivore design, or not totally of a carnivore design. We have grasping hands, most all primates that have a grasping hands are vegetarian. Our teeth are also of a more fruitarian design. I believe we are more of an omnivore design, meaning we can eat some meats but not too much.

Look at the rampant disease in this country; food is killing us! We all know it and see and hear about it everyday. Heart disease, Alzheimer's, strokes and diabetes... All come from high blood viscosity, from eating foods that make your blood thick. Eating mammalian meats, drinking milk and eating dairy products will increase blood viscosity! That's why going to a "thin blood" diet and reducing your intake of dairy products makes you naturally lose weight. But what else you lose is even greater. You will lose the disease process that occurs from eating lots of dairy products and animal, mammalian red meats. Good riddance! In return you will regain your health!

For weight loss, when you "trick" your body with pills, or you starve yourself, the weight you lose will come back. Tricking yourself into burning fat because it's the only option your body has because you are on a low carb diet, is also, in my opinion, not good. Sure you'll lose weight, but will it stay off? Is it healthy for you? Pills and fat burning substances are not the answer, many of these will put you into a sympathetic fight or flight response making you agitated and unable to sleep. Going on a low carb diet is not the answer either, for obvious reasons.

A low blood viscosity diet, with poly-unsaturated fats and mono-unsaturated fats instead of saturated fats as much as possible, will make you healthier. Eating fewer (or no) mammalian eats, by abstaining or eating more fish, will make you healthier. Eating less dairy and not drinking milk, will make you lose weight, feel better, and be healthier.

Why do I say that 85% of people will lose weight on the Kiso Diet™? Some folks are already skinny and don't need to lose weight. To have heart disease, it does not matter how skinny you are! Those who can eat anything and not gain weight can still develop the plaque in their arteries that causes heart attacks and strokes. Just being skinny does not safe guard you against atherosclerosis if you eat a high blood viscosity diet! Those of you who are overweight to any degree will lose weight on the Kiso Diet™ for just following the Kiso Diet™ principles. What are the Kiso Diet™ principles you ask...here you go:

The fifteen commandments...

1. Stop eating and drinking anything but water or herbal tea 3 to 4 hours before going to bed.

2. Follow the 80% rule; when you are 80% full, stop eating!

3. Put small portions on your plate. If you pile lots of food on your plate, you will eat more. Also, you won't waste food this way.

4. Chew your food a lot. They say up to 100 times, but just try to chew your food completely.

5. Eat only a small amount of processed foods, bought only from the health food store, and eat them before 3 p.m. to give yourself plenty of time to burn it off.

6. Never, I mean never, have sodas. They are all bad. Limit yourself to one cup of store-bought juice per day because drinking more can lead to too much sugar in your diet.

7. Don't eat fried foods at all. If you absolutely can't avoid them, take off the fried parts. For example, if you have to eat fried chicken, take off the fried skin. Don't eat any chips! Even chips made with "no trans fatty acids," are still made with oil.

8. Use milk substitutes in your coffee or on your cereal. I love the new coconut milk coffee or tea creamers. Find the products you like and use them!

9. Only eat 3 eggs per week, total. It can be all at once or one every once in awhile. Eggs are high in cholesterol and saturated fats. If you want an omelet, go ahead, but only once a week!

10. If you must have sugar in your coffee, then only have it once a day. Better yet, try a "natural" sugar alternative like Stevia or agave, that doesn't cause the rise in blood sugar that sugar does.

11. If you want to lose weight, even a little weight, eat one meal a day from the blender. A smoothie in place of a meal is a good way to get nutrition, plus it's easy to digest and it can give you the fresh fruits you need everyday.

12. Only drink two ounces of alcohol a day. That's two small glasses of wine, or two shots of hard liquor. Beer is laden with calories and can make you gain weight quickly, so is not a recommended alcohol to drink...sorry.

13. No drinking milk! No, No, No. Milk is bad for your body. It's just bad. Chipmunks don't drink cat milk and monkeys don't drink human milk. Humans are not designed to digest human breast milk after the age of two, and we're not designed to digest animal milk at all, EVER.

14. Eat cheese sparingly, with consciousness! I love cheese, but it does have saturated fat and can contain hormones and toxins if it's non organic. Buy organic cheese, flavor soups, salads, and pasta with it, but don't over do it!

15. Don't eat mammalian meats, or at least abstain 90% of the time. Shrimp and shellfish are not recommended because of toxins and high cholesterol.

Moving on...

The biggest other reason for losing weight on the Kiso Diet™...Exercise!

Following the Kiso Diet™ you will be exercising and the great thing about exercise is that it will increase your tonus. What is tonus? It's the muscle tone of your body. The more your body is toned, the more it increases your metabolism! Increasing your metabolism helps you lose weight all day long and all night long.

When you exercise, you burn the glycogen in your muscles and liver. This allows the sugar that's been eaten and stored as glycogen to enter your muscles (a process facilitated by insulin), instead of being converted to fat down the road. So when you do have a sweet, fat is burned up instead of making its way into your fat cells. Yes, sugar can eventually be stored as "fat". So it's not just fat that's stored as fat, but sugar can become stored as fat as well. This process is lessened the more you work out. Why? Because as you begin to work out INSULIN activity basically shuts down, and stays down, for the duration of your exercise. This allows you to burn both the fat in your blood and the stored fat in your body.

Exercise in the morning before eating anything! You can burn up to three times more body fat by exercising in the morning.

Exercising in the morning... A huge concept for fat loss!

Why exercise in the morning? Why does it burn up to three times more fat? In the Kiso Diet™ you are not supposed to eat for 3 to 4 hours before going to bed. If you sleep for eight, you've gone 12 hours without eating. It's the time you have the least amount of insulin present in your blood. That's precisely why your doctor has you go 12 hours without eating when fasting for a glucose test. Your glycogen stores are very low. Why is glucose stored anyway?

Your body stores glucose for fuel. It primarily stores it in your liver and your muscles. Remember I stated that the preferred fuel in your body is carbohydrates, and carbs come from carbohydrate foods and sugars? After you have eaten some carbs, it's stored as glucose. In order to store glucose in the muscles, you need insulin. That's where insulin comes into play in your body.

Have you ever heard of carbohydrate loading? Or carb loading? It's what marathoners do before a big running event. They eat pastas and other complex carbohydrates days before a big run. That way, when the big day comes, they've got tons of energy stored as glycogen in their muscles and in their livers. They can go much longer because of these "carbo stores" that are there for extra energy. Marathoners don't want to store fat. Why? Because fats are harder to burn and you have to "go through" the glycogen stores first. Plus glycogen gives you lots of energy and the burning of this energy is clean.

Remember the analogy of diesel fuel compared with regular gas compared with propane? Yes, glycogen is the cleanest fuel for your body and is like burning propane!

If you wake up and you just can't get going, now is the time to drink your coffee or tea, or better yet, green tea (lots of anti-oxidants). Try drinking it without sugar. If you must sweeten it, use Stevia or agave. But believe it or not, one teaspoon full of sugar is only 16 calories and is burned up pretty quickly if you exercise but causes an insulin spike stopping the release of fat from fat stores.   So avoid pure sugar!

With exercise, because insulin release is halted, your fat stores are burned depending on the amount of aerobic force you put into your workouts. The reason walking is such a good tool for losing weight is that your fat is efficiently burned when your body is moving at about 60% of your maximum heart rate. This is actually better for fat burning than working out at 70%! If you exercise too hard, you by-pass the fat burning that happens at 60% of maximum heart rate, and start getting into the protein burning stage at 70 to 80% of your maximum heart rate. Working out at this harder rate will tear down your muscles and will build your actual muscle strength later, but for those wanting to burn fat, keep in "the zone"!

What happens if you can't get up in the morning to work out either because you're tired (you'll get used to waking up and working out, believe me), or because of time constraints? You can do your aerobic workout later in the day after weight lifting.

Because weight lifting burns the glycogen stores in your muscles, after you lift weights with the various muscle groups of your body, your body has no choice but to go to the second gas tank, your fat stores in your body. Any exercise will do this because of the drop in insulin that takes place when you exercise! So if you cannot workout as soon as you get up, you can go to a gym in the day (or work out at home) and then weight lift first, burning the glycogen out of your muscles, then do your aerobic work out either on a machine (like an elliptical trainer or treadmill), or by walking or jogging. You can also do them at the same time. Doing an *aerobics class* with **weights** is a way to *deplete your glycogen stores*, as well as *sustain your heart rate*. There are lots of good classes or DVDs (Gilad's are wonderful!) to follow that will burn your glycogen stores and give you an aerobic workout, burning the fat stored in your body.

Other reasons for working out in the morning:

Besides your insulin level being at its lowest, getting your workout out of the way is great. You don't have to worry about when you can workout during the day 'cause you've already done it!

Endorphin rush! Yes, when you workout in the morning when your stored glycogen is low, you get a bigger endorphin rush. Endorphins are an opiate-like substance and are released when you exercise for longer periods of time. They are released after about 30 minutes of sustained aerobic activity.

Endorphins are good for your mood and can last quite a while, making you feel better during the day. Because it's an opiate-like substance, it's said to also kill pain during the day. So if you work out in the morning and get your endorphins released, you will likely feel less pain during the day in your body. That means if you have a sore joint or joints in your body, they'll feel better for most of the day, after your morning work out.

Increase in metabolism is another reason to work out, period! After you work out, your body's metabolic rate rises. It stays elevated for hours after you work out. If you work out in the morning, you have a higher metabolism for the hours during the day while you are carrying out your normal activities. If you work out at night, you only have a few hours to put your higher metabolism to work for you. Why? Because when you go to bed, your metabolic rate shuts down. So you'll get the biggest weight loss benefit from working out in the morning. The earlier you work out in the day, the better off you are for metabolism's sake. But if weight it not an issue or you are over 50 years of age, it's often easier on your body to work out at night. Why? Because your body has been warmed up already and you are less likely to injure yourself working out at night compared to the morning when, as you get older, the body is stiffer. That's why doing yoga is nice at night. It's a more yin exercise and you're stretching. Stretching is great! But it is often when you do pull a muscle. So always warm up, jog a few minutes or jump up and down or do jumping jacks just to warm yourself up before beginning to stretch.

By the way, using lighter weights is aerobic too. Generally, exercising with heavy weights is an anaerobic activity meaning it tears down the muscle tissue by depriving it of oxygen. This anaerobic exercise is what body builders use because this "tearing down" of the muscle is precisely what makes the muscle "build up" afterwards. But by using light weights when exercising, you keep breathing. When you lift heavy weights, you hold your breath momentarily as you lift, which makes it anaerobic. On the other hand, lifting light weights and "breathing" the whole time makes this exercise an aerobic activity. Because you're not using "heavy" weights, you will injure yourself much less.

A note about breathing... Closing your mouth when you breathe while working out, aids in making you more relaxed. The old fight or flight response kicks in when you open your mouth wide when you breathe. Opening your mouth mimics what occurs when you are attacked. When attacked, you open your mouth to get as much air as you can before fighting or fleeing from your opponent (fleeing is much preferred!). So when doing exercise and trying to change from a person in sympathetic over-ride to a more balanced type person, i.e. keeping in touch with your parasympathetic nervous system, try breathing through your nose as much as possible. You can also breathe in through your nose and exhale through your mouth if breathing entirely through your nose is difficult.

Fat stores...

Let's talk about storing fat, or losing fat for that matter. Most of us know that fat is stored in your body in fat cells. But did you know that during your adolescent years, fat cells in your body can be added or taken away? The number of fat cells in your body is not permanently determined until around the age of 18. For example, if you are 9 years old and are very fat, you obviously have a lot of fat cells on your body. These fat cells can be shed until you are about the age of 18. Once you mature, your fat cells are there for good. This means that if you had lots of fat cells throughout your entire adolescent years and are now 19, you pretty much will always have the same amount of fat cells for the rest of your life (unless you get lipo surgery which reduces your fat cells, yikes!). That's why as you become an adult it's important to stay slim to keep fat stores to a minimum.

So let's say you have "fat stores," lots of them. These fat cells are with you for life, but they can be full of fat, or they can be empty. Feeding them saturated fats will inflate them. In fact there is a relationship between cellulite and saturated fat. As I have mentioned before, saturated fat comes primarily from either mammalian meats or from dairy. So if you want to see your cellulite go away, the Kiso Diet™ will help do this for sure.

OK, so how does the Kiso Diet™ naturally make you lose weight? Glad you asked.

Following this diet you don't have to deprive yourself of good tasting food or sacrifice your wants and desires eating bland food that just doesn't hit the spot. There's no need for that.

Because the Kiso Diet™ does not have much in the way of saturated fats, you can safely eat good fats like olive oil, flax seed oil, avocados, nuts, fish oil etc. You can have flax oil on your salad and you can cook with the "good" oils too. Most mono-unsaturated and polyunsaturated fats are good fats and actually do some nice things for you. Just look at the Italian culture and its people. They are healthy in spite of the fact that they actually eat dairy and animal fats. But they do two things that we also do on the flexitarian side of Kiso Diet™ that help them; they cook with olive oil and eat fish.

Olive oil and most mono-unsaturated fats help reduce inflammation in the body. They are good for asthma and arthritis too. Mono-unsaturated fats are also good for increasing the good HDL cholesterol and decreasing the bad LDL cholesterol. Use extra virgin olive oil, it's the highest form of olive oil available. Don't over heat olive oil when cooking, and store it in a dark sealed bottle so it won't go bad. You can also find mono-unsaturated fats in avocados, canola oil, peanut oil, sunflower oil and sesame seed oil.

Poly-unsaturated fats have the essential fatty acids, or EFAs and DHAs, I talked about earlier. Remember, the omega 3s are golden, omega 3 fatty acids do things like reduce inflammation, keep blood from excessive clotting, reduce cholesterol and triglycerides in the blood, decrease blood thickness and have also been shown to prevent the growth of cancer cells.

While the complete affects of eating foods high in omega 3 are not fully known, some sources also say it can prevent depression, aid in cardiovascular health overall, improve infant cognitive development, as well as prevent osteoporosis and eye disease.

Here is an expanded list of foods containing omega 3s. Flaxseeds are the highest! Then the following:

- Walnuts
- Soybeans
- Brussels Sprouts
- Cauliflower
- Tofu
- Cabbage
- Shrimp
- Salmon
- Herring
- Sardines
- Anchovies
- Snapper
- Halibut
- Other freshwater fish

Omega 6s, which also fall in the category of poly-unsaturated fatty acids, are numerous in our American diet.

Basically meat is high in omega 6 EFAs. Omega 6s tend to increase inflammation.

Most omega 6 fatty acids in the diet come from vegetable oils as linoleic acid (LA). Linoleic acid is converted to gamma-linolenic acid (GLA) in the body. It is then further broken down to arachidonic acid (AA). To a great extent, omega 6s are found primarily in processed foods!

The ratio of omega 3 to omega 6 is an important factor. Our standard American diet provides us with a ratio of about 1 omega 3 to 18 omega 6, that is way out of balance! We should strive to have a balance of 1 (omega 3) to 5 (omega 6). This would be optimum. How can you do this?

Don't eat too much in the way of processed foods. Eat mostly whole foods. Eating crackers, cookies and other processed foods will definitely push you into the inflammation range and out of balance. If you do eat processed foods, make sure they came from the health food store to guarantee you that you won't be getting your omega 6s from GM sources. Corn and its evil offshoot high fructose corn syrup are the most used GM products sold in the world today. GM corn is feed to non-organically raised livestock, GM high fructose corn syrup is found in most processed foods. So eating meats and processed foods from a regular grocery store is a good way to ingest GM food products into your body. Very bad stuff!

Chapter 17

Making the Kiso Diet™ Work for You

It's recommended that everyone starting the Kiso Diet™ begin with the Vegan portion for a one week period. This is essential for three reasons. The first reason is that buying food on a vegan diet takes expertise. Trying not to get any dairy or eggs is sometimes hard at first, but after one week, you will already be well on your way to figuring out how to eat on a vegan diet. The second reason is to change your tongue. Your tongue may be suited to the SAD diet and you will need a lesson in how a clean vegan diet tastes. Chances are you will start to see, right away, the beautiful textures and tastes while eating on a vegan diet. The third reason is for cleansing. A vegan diet is very cleansing and one week will do a great job at cleansing your body.

The second week of the Kiso Diet can be centered on a lacto-ovo vegetarian diet. You will find this diet much easier to live on than the vegan diet. You will have more leeway on what to buy on this diet. You've already gotten used to a vegan diet for one week and you may opt to stay on that vegan diet for a few more weeks, or even forever. But if you move to a lacto-ovo, low dairy vegetarian diet, you may be so satisfied you won't feel the need to go for the flexitarian diet.

On the third week, you can start eating flexitarian, if you are so inclined. See, you've already had a real life education on good diets, the vegan and the lacto-ovo, low dairy vegetarian diet. But without that prior, real life knowledge of what it's like to eat on the vegan and vegetarian diets, you would be unable to properly go on the flexitarian diet. Because remember, the flexitarian diet means that primarily you are a vegetarian, but occasionally have fish or fowl. In order for you not to contaminate your flexitarian diet, you have to know how to eat as a vegan and as a vegetarian to properly carry out a flexitarian lifestyle.

So, as we get into the food buying coming up next, just remember, you're starting out on the vegan part of the diet and this will require you to buy foods with NO dairy or animal products at all. In order to do this, you must read labels and make choices that follow this plan. Of course, if you move to the lacto-ovo vegetarian diet and eventually to the flexitarian diet, your shopping will become easier.

Shopping...

Shopping on the Kiso Diet™ is easy. If fact it's easier than shopping for your old diet. How do we shop on the Kiso Diet? It's funny, but when you go into a grocery store, whether it's a health food store or a big chain grocery store, most of the good foods are out on the perimeter of the store. Try this: when you enter the store, go to the right. You'll probably find the whole grain breads and vegetables there, then you'll progress into the fish and fowl areas.

On the Kiso Diet™, we aren't buying much in the way of processed foods. This means both processed meats and processed foods in general. Don't eat processed foods from a general grocery store, unless they are healthy processed foods that you're eating as your snack during the day, once a day, at an appropriate time for you. (These days, regular grocery stores carry health foods, so sometimes you can find trusted health food snacks there.)

The inside or middle of the grocery store has all the sodas and processed junk foods. It also has canned foods, which you should avoid as much as possible because unless they are organic canned food, even then don't eat them daily. Canned foods have much less life force energy compared to home cooked foods. It's made in a factory where no one cares and it's been sitting in the can forever. This goes for most frozen foods as well, though frozen vegetables and frozen whole fruits aren't too bad so they are allowed.

On the Kiso Diet™, do not eat frozen dinners or frozen desserts and canned foods very often, they are all dead. You will be making your food selections from fresh whole foods as often as possible.

Frozen and canned foods are convenient. That's why they appeal to so many people. Some canned foods are occasionally OK to buy like beans for Mexican foods, but buy from the health food store as much as possible. You can also find packaged, already prepared foods in packages ready to be heated up in hot water. These are far better and still contain some of the life force and energy inherent to fresh whole foods. They make great Indian cuisine that's scrumptious!

When you enter the inside or *center* areas of a store, just get what you need. You can head for things like boxed soymilk or other types of milk substitutes. Get your whole beans. Buy fresh, organic juices if you like, but limit your consumption to one glass a day (as mentioned before). Avoid the grocery store's dairy areas that have yogurt and milk. At the health food store, you can buy soy yogurts, which are very good. You can even buy soy cheeses, which aren't bad at all. They take a bit of time to get used to, but you will acquire a taste for them. If you buy Asian food you must be careful not to get MSG (monosodium glutamate) in your products. Kim Chee and hot sauces are often heavily laden.

Buying your staples for the Kiso Diet™

Let's talk about the staples, or the base of what you will be having at every meal. I will list four. Two are whole foods and preferred, and two are "processed" whole foods.

Rice (a whole food)

That's our number one staple on the Kiso Diet™. I hear many people say they stay away from rice because it's a starch and that's not good on a low carb diet. Rice is essential on the Kiso Diet™. Let me rephrase that: **brown** rice is essential on the Kiso Diet™.

Let's talk about yin and yang again. The outside of the skin on anything is yang and the inside, soft part is yin. The yang skin, holds the fruit or potato or grain together. This outer skin is where most of the vitamins are. It's not as sweet as the inside but is absolutely necessary when eating on the Kiso Diet™. You will get use to eating the skin or husk of the rice in a short amount of time.

If you only eat the yin, or the inside, of all your fruits and vegetables, you will only get the part that is sugary. If you only eat white rice, you will indeed get too much starch, which will turn to sugar in your body. But if you eat that starch with the husk or skin of the rice or potato, you will slow down the process of digestion. This in itself will slow down the insulin poured out from your pancreas in response to a sugar in your blood stream. So in the Kiso Diet™, we always cook the whole food, that means skin and all, when cooking something.

Brown rice has tons of nutrients and tons of fiber. It's good stuff and the bulk of it in your stomach helps you feel full quickly. There are different types of brown rice that you can choose from:

Sweet brown rice is usually bought only at the health food store. It's so sweet, it almost tastes like white rice, and it's available in many forms.

There is the regular brown rice, which many people love and acquire a taste for. It's very hard and nutty. If you have a good rice cooker, you will have a setting on your machine that cooks brown rice longer making it softer and tastier than cooking brown rice quickly. If you under-cook brown rice, it can be hard when you have a bite of it.

Then there is brown basmati rice (Indian rice), which has a unique flavor. I love it. Some folks mix half brown rice with half white rice in order to make it softer and more palatable. Some people do this for a while until they get use to the total brown rice texture.

Using a rice cooker for brown rice is almost necessary. I say almost because you can cook brown rice in a pot on the stove, but it comes out hard. If you've ever made white rice in a pot on the stove, you know it turns out quite well. But cooking brown rice in a pot does not come out as well, it's usually hard and kind of dry. Brown rice cooked in a rice cooker, especially a newer rice cooker with a brown rice setting, comes out soft and fluffy, perfect every time. It tastes and looks similar to white rice, especially if you use what is known as sweet brown rice from the health food store. It is still brown rice, it still has the hull on the rice, but it's more broken down compared with brown rice cooked in a pot on the stove. It's very tasty!

Whether you make the rice on the stove or in a rice cooker, you must measure out the rice. Usually one cup of rice, to two cups of water. Then you must wash the rice, rinsing it 3 or 4 times. White rice has a kind of powder in it that must be washed out completely. Now put the pot on the stove or set your rice cooker timer. Of course if you have a rice cooker timer, it will automatically shut off. If you are cooking it on the stove, you first boil the rice and water, then drop the heat to about 3 (or low) for another 20 minutes. I used to make fantastic rice doing this for many years when I was young.

Potatoes (a whole food)

Potatoes are essential for variety on the Kiso Diet™. There are so many types of potatoes! All are excellent choices, but be mindful of the manner in which they're prepared. Remember to cut the eyes out of the potato, as there are toxins in the eyes. Always wash potatoes well and cook them with the skins on.

Potatoes can be prepared in many different ways. Boil them and mash them afterwards, skins and all, with a bit of good margarine (no saturated or trans fatty acids) and soymilk. Or wrap them in foil and bake for about 45 minutes at 375 degrees. Eat the whole baked potato, skin too! Make potato skins by cutting the potato in half and after baking, scooping out the center and mashing with good margarine, or a bit of olive oil. Return the mixture to the skins and top with some cheese, onions, salsa, or a non-dairy sour cream alternative (try tofutti). It's all good!

Pasta (a processed food)

Pasta is another staple on the Kiso Diet. It's not a whole food, so should not be eaten every day, but it's fine to eat up to twice a week. It has a good glycemic index and does not spike insulin. You can also buy whole grain pasta, which tastes different than traditional pasta; kind of like the difference between whole unbleached wheat bread and white bread. Of course white bread is much worse than regular pasta as it uses bleach to make it white. Pasta, even traditional pasta, is much healthier than any white bread. Pasta actually has a low glycemic index rate, so it does not cause an insulin spike.

There are basically two types of pasta. **Pasta** is a generic term for <u>noodles</u> made from unleavened dough of either wheat or buckwheat flour. Pastas include varieties like ravioli and tortellini that are filled with other ingredients.

Pasta comes in hundreds of different shapes: spaghetti, which are thin strings; macaroni, which are tubes; fusilli, which are corkscrew spirals; lasagna, which come in sheets; and more. The shape doesn't affect the nutritional value, nor does whether it's fresh or dried. If the pasta is dried, it can last up to two years on the shelf! If it's fresh, it should be eaten within one day. When eating pasta, always have a non meat pasta sauce. White sauces are a no-no, due to too much milk and cream. Get a good organic red pasta sauce for sure.

Breads (a processed food)

Breads

Breads are a natural part of the Kiso Diet™. Whole food breads are the only kind to buy. Whole food breads are made without artificial colors, flavors, sweeteners, preservatives or trans fats.

Bread staples on the Kiso Diet™ include whole wheat bread and all its types, like oat bread, flaxseed bread, honey wheat bread, etc. There are many kinds of bread that we often forget about like cornbread, focaccia, bagels, and croissants. Then there are the flat breads, like pitas or pocket breads. These are Middle Eastern breads made by steaming. The steam puffs up the bread, then when it cools it becomes flat, leaving bubbles or pockets. They're great for stuffing with things like falafel, vegetables, and fish, for that matter. Get the whole wheat variety, for sure. Naan breads from India are also flat but have no pockets. They're often available with added ingredients like onion, which are so good! Eating plain naan bread with Indian lentil beans is my favorite.

Tortillas are absolutely useful on the Kiso Diet™. You can wrap things in them like different vegetables, beans, onions and avocados. They come in many styles nowadays, like spinach and tomato just to name a few.

On the Kiso Diet™, food items outside of the four staples are considered side dishes. Side dishes will provide your protein.

Getting protein

Try different types of protein. Whether or not you are a vegetarian, vegan or flexitarian, try protein-laden foods like beans, nuts, seeds, peas, tofu and soy products. These foods will give you new options at meal-time and at snack time.

• Beans: black beans, navy beans, garbanzos, and lentils are good options.

• Nuts: almonds, walnuts, pistachios, and pecans are great choices.

• Soy products: try tofu, soymilk, tempeh, and veggie burgers.

There is also one more tasty meat alternative that you can make a variety of dishes with. It's called seitan. It's made from wheat gluten. (If you are gluten intolerant, don't eat this.) It tastes very much like meat and is loaded with protein. We will show a recipe later!

Beans

Beans are heavy in protein, but the protein is not a whole protein. In other words, beans are missing a few amino acids, which can be supplied by the rest of the food on your plate. So even though beans don't have all the amino acids to make a whole protein, combining them with the amino acids from your brown rice makes beans' proteins whole! (Or combine beans with your bread, or what ever else you choose for your staple.) There are many, many kinds of beans.

Lentils are great and are often used in Indian cuisine. There are many different types. Some are darker, some light, you can experiment with different dishes. Lentils are very high in protein.

Pinto beans are a favorite in Mexican food and are used in chili, they can also be put on top of your salad. Very delicious. I love to cook chili beans with a meat substitute that looks like ground beef. Honestly, I've made chili with beans in a pressure cooker and it turned out incredible.

White beans or navy beans (used in the Navy long ago) are very good and can be cooked in so many ways. You can make baked beans out of them, in fact most commercial baked beans are made with navy beans.

Prepared beans freeze well, so you can cook your beans in advance and put them in a bag to freeze. Then when you want to eat them, simply thaw and heat as needed. Bean burgers are also a great source of protein and very tasty, having a meaty like texture and flavor.

Nuts

Nuts are a very high in fiber, they are also high in fat but very high in protein. They have insoluble dietary fiber (cellulose), in the skin. Their oils are composed primarily of unsaturated fatty acids, they are a great source of vitamin E. Nuts are high in fat, but acceptable on the Kiso Diet™, because it's a naturally lower fat diet. You can eat nuts daily if you like, as a healthy snack. They do contain saturated fat, but a good form of saturated fat that does not promote atherosclerosis in the way that meat fat does.

Nuts are an excellent source of B vitamins. Plain raw or roasted nuts are low in sodium but salted nuts are high in salt so try to eat the unsalted variety.

What's in nuts?

One half cup of dry roasted unsalted almonds has eight grams of dietary fiber. It has about 36 g total of total fat but only 2.7 g of saturated fat. The fat breakdown goes like this: 23.2 g monounsaturated, 8.7 g polyunsaturated. That's not bad at all! Nuts, being plant foods, have no cholesterol at all.

Soy products: Try tofu! We will show you a recipe for miso soup later and a tofu dish too. Tofu is huge in the orient and it will blend itself into any dish. Because it's bland, it seems to enhance a spicy dish just right.

Tempeh is a traditional food of Japan and Indonesia. Soy is fermented in a process that binds soybeans into a cake form. It's used in soups and eaten with rice and is very tasty!

Veggie soy burgers are a great source of protein and help the variety factor in the Kiso Diet™. Even if you are on the flexitarian part of the Kiso Diet™, veggie burgers give you the option of eating a hamburger (without the meat) and getting the full enjoyment of it!

Vegetables that go with your staples are numerous. Vegetables can be eaten raw, boiled, steamed, baked, or even roasted. I love having a veggie kabob cooked on an open fire.

Squash

You can make pumpkin, which is a favorite in Japanese cooking. It's looks different than your Halloween variety pumpkin, is very tasty and goes great with rice or in a soup. Squash in general are divided into summer and winter, but all can be eaten and are very delicious. All parts of the squash can be eaten. Favorite varieties are zucchini, yellow squash, long squash, short round ones... there many types and varieties. Try them all.

Stir fry vegetables are recommended once or twice a week.

Hard vegetables like zucchini, sweet peppers, spinach and mung bean sprouts, can be quickly stir-fried at high heat without the addition of extra liquid, because they are high moisture vegetables.

Vegetables that require more cooking time are denser, low moisture vegetables like broccoli and carrots. Most recipes call for the vegetables to be stir-fried briefly and then boiled in a liquid such as chicken broth or a vegetable broth.

Another option is to briefly blanch the vegetables prior to stir-frying.

Lots of vegetables fall somewhere in between these two extremes. Two very popular stir fry veggies are snow peas and asparagus. They have medium moisture, but are thick at the same time. They are traditional veggies in Chinese cuisine.

You can even add a kind of Chinese pasta to your stir fry. These Chinese noodles are very tasty and absorb the spices used to prepare the meal.

There are a few types to try. Wheat noodles made with or without egg are the most often used and can be fried or stir fried.

Rice noodles, made from rice flour, salt, and water, can be thick or thin, and have a clear consistency. These noodles are usually stir fried, or try adding them to plain miso soup to liven it up!

Soups are recommended once or twice a week!

Vegetable soups are so satisfying. You can have them with the bread of your choice. Again, it's whole foods, bradah, so no worries. We will give you a few recipes for soups coming up. You can also put chicken or turkey in the soups if you are practicing the flexitarian diet. Soup can be low in fat and high in good carbs and protein!

Miso soups are great, there are many different kinds but they usually have something very beneficial in them besides tofu for protein, it's seaweed! Seaweeds are very good for you and putting them into your miso soup is an easy way to get them.

Wakame is usually sold in dried form, and is soaked in water before you use it in your soups. The taste is light and very good.

Kombu is a large type of seaweed that is often used as a soup stocks such as nabe. Nabe is a soup with all kinds of stuff in it. In Japan, they put fish or chicken in it as well as mushrooms.

Nori are thin, dried seaweed sheets. Nori sheets are used in many sushi dishes, for rice balls and my kids love to eat it plain!

Japanese mushrooms and mushrooms in general are very beneficial for health. They enhance all kinds of dishes from salads to sautés and are used traditionally in many Japanese dishes and soups. Very popular mushrooms found in Japanese cooking are the Shiitake, Maitake, Matsutake and Bunashimeji. Try them all!

Salads

Salads, made primarily of different types of lettuce are not to be heated up 'cause the vitamin C in the different lettuces will be killed upon heating (not to mention the lettuce wilts). That's why salads are eaten cold. The more colorful the salad, the more antioxidants there are.

Having salads in winter is not a good idea if you live in a cold climate. Salads are suited for a warm time of year. If you live in a cold area, having a cold salad is ill advised. I live in Hawaii, so I can have salads any time I want! Not to rub it in, but it does matter where you live. If you live in N. Dakota and it's the dead of winter, eat warm foods (something cooked) more often than cold, un-cooked vegetables. Those on a raw food diet, beware. Cold, raw foods are yin, yin, yin and very cooling for the body. If you are a vata type, which tends to be cold, then a raw food diet, in my opinion, can cause great harm. If folks eat salads too often, their joints begin to ache, it's true. It's a symptom of eating too much raw food.

Salads can be Greek, Italian, American, anything you can think of. Using vegetable oils like olive or flaxseed are advised as opposed to milk dressings like ranch. Always eat organic vegetables and wash them well. Washing your veggies with a vegetable wash from your health food store is advised. You can throw stuff in there to go with your lettuce like olives, dates, pine nuts, raisins, and even flowers! The sky's the limit.

Having cold pasta salads are one of my favorite things to eat for lunch!

Fish

We've all heard about toxins in fish; the big worry is mercury, from polluted waters. Women of childbearing age (15 to 44 years), pregnant women, nursing mothers and children under age 15 are the most susceptible to mercury poisoning. While mercury is a concern, fish offer some great nutritional benefits, making them an encouraged part of the Kiso Diet™.

So, which fish are safest to eat? Well, it's probably easier to tell you which fish **not** to eat and go from there.

FISH TO AVOID OR LIMIT YOUR CONSUMPTION OF:

Ocean fish:
Albacore (white) tuna; fresh, frozen or canned
King mackerel
Marlin
Shark
Spanish mackerel
Swordfish
Tilefish

Freshwater Fish:
Black crappie
Catfish (caught wild)
Jack fish (chain pickerel)
Largemouth bass (statewide)
Walleye from Lake Fontana and Lake Santeetlah (Graham and

Swain counties)
Yellow perch

If you're in a mercury high risk category, avoid the fish listed above. Other folks can safely enjoy fish two or three times a week without concern. Remember: Only buy fish that have been caught in the wild. Many farm raised fish are lower in mercury but will hurt you in other ways, so don't eat farm raised anything! They are often fed GM corn, which ruins the fish for human consumption.

Try to eat deep water, **oily fish.** Their fillets contain about 30 percent oil. This oil content seems high, but the oil is good for the heart and because the Kiso Diet™ is naturally low in oil, it's fine a few times a week. Examples include small fish like sardines, herring, and anchovy. Also larger fish like salmon, trout, and mackerel (King and Spanish mackerel have possible mercury, so be careful) are great.

Have fish with brown rice or wrap them in a pita bread with lettuce. Or try fish tacos. It's ono (that's DELICIOUS in Hawaiian)!

Fowl

Eating chicken or turkey is part of the flexitarian Kiso Diet™. Always buying organic, free range, no hormone fowl is the only way to go! As discussed earlier, fowl is high in omega

3 too, but should be heated up well over 180 degrees before eating. You can even buy uncured turkey and chicken meat to put into your sandwiches if you like. Eating an occasional turkey or chicken sausage is OK too.

What are some other things to make your taste buds more interested in your meals?

Pickles are great, but I'm talking about the Japanese varieties of pickles. They are called Tsukemono (pickled things) and are an everyday occurrence in a Japanese home. Some are made to be eaten within a few days, and some keep for a long time like traditional American pickles. The most common pickling vegetables are Chinese cabbage, regular cabbage, cucumbers, turnips and daikon radish. Some other kinds of vegetables used less commonly are carrots, celery, and various greens. Tsukemono are really good with ochazuke. This is a popular Japanese dish made with hot tea, rice and pickles. It's a very low cal snack or even can be a dinner or a meal replacement to enhance weight loss!

Another thing you can do is to cut and save the leaves from your vegetables and use them for garnish later. Instead of cutting the leaves off your celery, carrots, and daikon (Japanese white radish) you can chop them up and store them in the freezer and use them as garnish for your fish, fowl, and soups. It's very tasty indeed.

Of course you can replace a meal when on the weight loss portion of the Kiso Diet™ with a nice green drink or green drink smoothie as mentioned earlier.

Spice it up

When cooking on the Kiso Diet™ try many spices. Spices will help you not miss the meat found in every meal in the SAD American diet. You can use spices like: Basil, bay leaf, cilantro, chili pepper, clove, cumin, garlic, ginger, oregano, paprika, parsley, all kinds of peppers, Szechwan pepper, thyme, turmeric, wasabi, just to name a few.

For example, Thai and Indian cuisine taste fantastic because of all the spices they use in their cooking. Experimentation is the key and reading new recipes on line and trying new things is how you will get better at making your food taste better!

So there you go, you're on your way! Plan your meals every week, it makes it easy to shop. I always buy my veggies from the farmer's market (look for organic varieties), and from the health food store (look for organic and local). Big supermarket chains usually ship their vegetables from just a few sources. Making the journey takes time, so they usually harvest the vegetables too early, giving them a bland taste. Buying local vegetables is easy and they taste fresher.

Chapter 18

A New Way of Eating

It's nice to have an idea of what to eat every day on the Kiso Diet™. We will start with breakfast:

Breakfast menu

Breakfast sets the tone for the day. Exercise first, then reach for light, nutritious foods:

- Oatmeal, quick or whole or a mixture with oats.

- Smoothie, for a meal replacement loaded with your favorite nutrients.

- Cereals, with soymilk. It must be a whole grain cereal, only eaten once in awhile for variety. Cereal is not a whole food so it's not to be eaten every day.

- Miso soup. Great for the morning or evening.

- Bread of your choice with organic fruit on top or honey (local honey is better).

- Fruits. Fruits should be eaten first, alone because they don't mix well with other carbs or proteins. You can eat all kinds. Seasonal fruit is best. If it's summer or if you live in a warm climate, tropical fruits are wonderful. Papaya (non GMO, mostly strawberry papaya), pineapple, and bananas are tasty but have lots of sugar. Other great fruits are apples and oranges. See what's fresh at your grocer.

- Eggs. Only eat 3 eggs a week. So if you make a three egg omelets, do it just once a week. Have it with organic potatoes if you like.

A mid morning snack is fine. Try fruit, nuts, or a healthy baked treat like a whole grain muffin.

Lunch

- Lunch is usually a fast meal so quick or easily prepared items are nice like:

- Brown rice (all kinds) is the biggest staple on the Kiso Diet™ and should be eaten often. You can put anything with the brown rice you like. You can have cooked vegetables, beans, and fish or chicken if you like.

- Sandwiches of all kinds always use a mayonnaise substitute to cut down on the saturated fats of real mayonnaise.

- Having a meal replacement at lunch works well. I recommend a smoothie with your favorite additives.

- Salads are so good and satisfying at lunchtime. Eating a salad with dried tomatoes or pasta added helps to bulk up the salad for taste and to make it more substantial. Of course adding fish or chicken is an option on the flexitarian portion of the Kiso Diet.

- Burritos, tacos and Mexican food, and Southwest foods utilizing the tortilla are great for lunch. You can have them vegetarian or with meat. Avoid hard taco shells because of the fat content.

- Soups like a tomato bisque or a minestrone soup are nice at lunch. There are literally hundreds of soup combos.

- Veggie wraps are great. Again you are utilizing the tortilla, or try a pita bread sandwich. You can put hummus in there or make a falafel pita sandwich! Recipe later...

Mid afternoon snack on fruit, nuts, or a cookie from the health food store, even a piece of dark chocolate!

Dinner

Dinner is the best time for a larger meal with protein, since the quiet time after dinner allows you to digest. Remember to aim for at least three whole foods:

- Brown rice and fish or chicken can be eaten if on the flexitarian side of the diet. You can have brown rice with sautéed vegetables. You can have rice and beans, a great combination! All whole foods.

- Stir fried vegetables. Chinese and Japanese recipes as well as Thai recipes are fantastic! Recipes later...

- Pasta is a quick and delightful dinner to come home to or to make right after work. Have it with your bread of choice. There are so many kinds of pasta, you can experiment as you go along. For example, you can have lasagna with a meat replacement for ground beef. It's really taste and healthy too.

- A veggie burger with a soy patty or a bean patty is great. Making it like a regular hamburger, but without the added saturated fats of a beef burger!

- Soup! You can make all kinds of soups. Soups are a key dinner for any vegetarian diet. They're satisfying and good for you. Soups are low in fat and high in taste. Have soup with a good whole grain bread of choice.

- Indian food or Thai food vegetarian style is a key dinner in a flexitarian or vegetarian Kiso Diet. Dishes like dhal (a spiced lentil bean dish), or a masala curry dish with naan bread are oh so tasty. We will show you a few recipes and pictures of this!

- Mexican food made with all organic materials is good for you if you cut down on the cheese and replace the refried beans with organic 100% vegetarian black or refried beans. You can make anything from tamales to burritos.

These are just a few dishes to start with. You can add to your repertoire as time goes on. I believe this, and the recipes to follow will keep you busy for a while!

RECIPES

Visit our web site, kisodiet.com for photographs of these dishes, plus lots of other great recipes!

Rice Balls

Prepare steamed rice.

• Wash hands well, and put 2 pinches of salt in your slightly wet hand. Rub your hands to spread salt evenly in your hands.

• Put some warm rice in your hand and make a ball with a little pressure. (Use warm rice in order to make a nice shaped ball easily, but be careful not to burn your hands with hot rice.)

• You can mix sesame seeds, seaweeds, or vegetable pickles with the rice, as you wish.

Celery Leaf Soup
Serves four

1 Tbsp olive oil
2 cups minced celery leaves
½ cup minced celery
½ cup minced onion
½ cup minced carrot
½ cup diced potato
½ cup small seashell pasta
1 clove garlic
1 Tbsp thyme
3 cubes vegetable broth
5 cups water
pinch of salt and black pepper to taste

Cooking method:

• Turn the heat up to about medium. Heat olive oil in a stew pan. Add garlic, cook stirring quickly until you can just start smelling the garlic fragrance.

• Add all vegetables into the pan, cook until they become soft, stirring occasionally.

• Add water, thyme, and bring to boil.

• Reduce heat and add vegetable broth, black pepper and salt to taste. Cook another 15 minutes to 20 minutes on low heat.

Potato skin salad recipe
Serves four

4 large organic potatoes
½ Japanese cucumber
¼ carrot
¼ apple
vegan or vegetable oil mayonnaise
yellow mustard, or any kind of mustard
black pepper and salt to taste

Cooking Method:

• Wash potatoes well, and eliminate potato eyes and greenish colored skin.

• Bake potatoes for 40-45 minutes at 400 degrees.

• Meanwhile, cut cucumber, carrot and apple, and massage them with a pinch of salt. Set to the side.

• Place the baked potatoes in a large bowl, and mash with a fork.

• While the potatoes are hot, add the vegetables, mayonnaise, mustard, black pepper and salt to taste.

Serve warm, or cooled.

Stir Fried Vegetables
Serves two

1 Tbsp Olive oil
3 cups mixed vegetables, chopped thin
1 tsp ginger, finely chopped
1 tsp garlic, finely chopped
1 Tbsp soy sauce
1 Tbsp sake
1 Tbsp brown sugar
2-3 pinches white pepper or black pepper
1 pinch salt, or according to taste
¼ cup seaweed or vegetable broth
1 Tbsp Sesame Oil
Roasted sesame seeds

Cooking Method:

• Heat olive oil in a wok. Keep the flame medium.

• Add ginger and garlic. Stir. Add onions. Stir for 2 minutes.

• Add the rest of vegetables.

• Add soy sauce, sake, broth, pepper, brown sugar, and salt to taste. Mix, Keep aside.

• Add 1 Tbsp of water if you want to cook the vegetables soft.

• When the vegetables are almost fully cooked, add the roasted sesame seeds and sesame oil. Mix well to coat all the vegetables. Remove from heat and serve immediately.

Serve hot on a bed of plain steamed rice or noodles along with a salad of your choice.

Lemon curry stir-fried rice with fiber
Serves 2

½ cup onion, chopped thin
½ tomatoes, chopped thin
1 tsp ginger, finely chopped
1 tsp garlic, finely chopped
½ cup vegetable skin (carrot, celery, etc.)
¼ cup seaweed or vegetable broth
2 Tbsps lemon curry powder
1 tsp cumin seeds
1 Tbsp olive oil
1 pinch salt, or according to taste
2-3 pinches white or black pepper
chopped parsley, optional

Cooking Method:

• Prepare 3 bowls of Brown rice

• Heat olive oil in a wok. Keep the flame medium.

• Add ginger, garlic and cumin seeds. Stir until you can just start smelling their fragrance.

• Add onions. Stir for 2 minutes.

• Add the vegetable skin, and lemon curry powder.

• Add broth and brown rice.

• Add salt and pepper to taste.

Sprinkle parsley on the top, serve.

Seitan
Serves 2

1 (8 ounce) package seitan
1/3 cup nutritional yeast
1 tsp garlic powder
1tsp thyme
1/8 tsp ground black pepper
1/3 cup soy sauce
2 Tbsps tamari
2 Tbsps vegetable oil

Cooking Method:

• In a small bowl, combine the nutritional yeast, garlic powder, thyme, and black pepper.

• In another small bowl, combine soy sauce and tamari.

• Dip the seitan strips in the soy tamari mixture, then in the yeast and spice mixture. Set aside.

• Heat oil in a skillet over medium heat. Fry seitan in batches until browned on all sides.

Serve as meat replacement in any dish, or with noodles, rice or potatoes.

Miso soup
Serves 2

2 cups water
1 Tbsp fish broth or seaweed broth (dashi)
¼ tsp sake
¼ tsp soy sauce
2 - 3 Tbsps miso paste
¼ cup cubed sweet potatoes
1 Tbsp dry seaweed (wakame)
1 Tbsp minced green onion

Cooking method:

• Put the dashi and water in a large sauce pan over high heat, bring to boil.

• Add sake and soy sauce.

• Add the sweet potatoes and dry seaweed.

• Simmer until the potatoes become soft (when a chopstick will go through), turn off the heat.

• Dip a ladle into the pot, capturing some broth. Slowly melt the miso paste in the ladle with the broth. When fully dissolved, add miso to pot. (Because the miso paste dissolves slowly, you can't just throw the miso paste into the pan without dissolving it this way, or it turns bitter.)

• Make sure the taste is OK, if you need more miso paste, you can add a little bit more, dissolving as above.

Garnish with chopped green onions.

Tofu Tacos
Serves 4

1 large onion, chopped
2 Tbsps olive oil
4 cloves garlic, finely diced
1 block (1 lb) firm tofu, rinsed & drained
1/2 cup tomato based pasta sauce (any kind)
1 tsp paprika
1 tsp cayenne pepper
1 tsp ground cumin
1 tsp season salt (or celery salt)
2 tsps dried oregano
1 cup fresh cilantro, chopped

Cooking method:

• In large saucepan over medium heat, cook onions in olive oil until golden brown (approx 5 mins), stirring frequently.

• Add garlic, cook until garlic begins to brown.

• Pat tofu on paper towel to press out excess moisture, then crumble into the pan (texture will look like scrambled eggs).

• Add pasta sauce and spices. Cook, stirring frequently, until most of liquid has cooked out.

• Add cilantro at end, stir in and serve. Garnish with your favorite taco accompaniments: grated cheese, tomatoes, avocado, and lettuce. Serve in soft tortillas.

Hint – scramble leftover tofu taco with an egg for breakfast!

Veggie Tortilla Wraps
Serves 4

4 tortillas
2 potatoes, cubed
1 tbsp green onion
1/4 yellow onion
1/4 bell pepper
1/4 mushrooms
2 Tbsps olive oil, separated
3 Tbsps pineapple salsa
1 Tbsp tofuy (sour cream)
salt and pepper to taste
cheese (optional)

Cooking method:

• Soak cubed potatoes in water for 5 minutes, drain, pat dry
• Heat oil in a skillet over medium heat
• Add potatoes, cook for 5 minutes on medium then turn to low heat and cover.
• Once in awhile, uncover to flip potatoes in order to cook all potatoes evenly
• Add salt and pepper to taste.
• When potatoes are completely cooked, remove from heat.
• In another fry pan, heat oil and cook all vegetables.
• Add salt and pepper to taste

Warm tortillas in the microwave, then place some potatoes, cooked vegetables, salsa, and sour cream on the tortilla. Sprinkle with cheese if desired. Wrap, and enjoy!

Spicy Black Beans
Serves 2

1 Tbsp olive oil
1 onion, chopped
4 cloves garlic, finely diced
1 15 oz can black beans, rinsed & drained
1 tsp chipotle chile peppers in adobo sauce (canned)
1/4 cup fresh cilantro, chopped

Cooking method:

• In saucepan over medium heat, cook onions in olive oil until golden brown (approx 5 mins), stirring frequently.

• Add garlic, cook until garlic begins to brown.

• Add beans and chipotle peppers, cook until beans are tender, approx 20 minutes.

• Add cilantro at end, stir in and serve.

Enjoy as a side dish, with rice for a main course, or in bean tacos.

Caution – chipotle chile peppers are HOT. If your tastes are mild, start with 1/2 tsp, add more to taste.

Cauliflower Curry
Serves 4

1 Tbsp olive oil
1 onion, chopped
2 tsps yellow curry powder
2 cups cauliflower, chopped in small florets
1 15 oz can garbanzo beans, rinsed & drained
1 10 oz can diced tomatoes with green chiles
1 14 oz can unsweetened coconut milk
1/4 cup fresh cilantro, chopped
Salt & pepper to taste

Cooking method:

• In large saucepan over medium heat, cook onions in olive oil until golden brown (approx 5 mins), stirring frequently.

• Add curry powder, stir for 20 seconds, then add beans and cauliflower. Stir and cook for 1 minute.

• Add tomatoes and coconut milk. Increase heat and bring to boil, cook at low boil, stirring occasionally, until beans are tender and liquid has thickened, about 20 minutes.

• Stir in cilantro, add salt and pepper to taste.

Serve with naan bread or chapattis (Indian flat bread).

Index

Acknowledgements

I wish to express my gratitude to T. Colin Campbell, Ph.D, for his ground-breaking research and hard work; and to John Robbins, who's written works inspired my early interest in dietary health.

I would like to thank Gilad for giving me the opportunity to speak at his fitness camps, and for showing me what exercise can do for us all.

And last, I owe a debt of gratitude to my patients for entrusting me with their care; allowing me to correlating high blood viscosity with joint problems, heart disease, and a myriad of other illnesses. This holopathogenetic association is essential to the Kiso Method's ability to relieve chronic pain and suffering, and inspired The Kiso Diet™.

About the Author

Dr. Craig Zion Cain was born in Long Beach, California and raised in Orange County. He did most of his undergraduate work in Stockton, California, before moving to the San Jose area to study at Palmer College of Chiropractic West, where he graduated in 1988 with a doctorate degree. He has practiced chiropractic in many areas in California including Santa Clara, Milpitas, San Jose, Monterey Bay and Los Gatos.

Over the years he studied multiple forms of healing arts; including Oriental Medicine, Japanese bodywork therapies and energy therapies. He holds several black belts in various martial arts from China, Japan and Vietnam. His interest in Asian arts took him to Japan, where he lived, worked and practiced for several years. He now makes his home on the Big Island of Hawaii.

Dr. Cain is the founder of Kiso Method™, a unique and entirely original healing technique taught worldwide to chiropractors, Asian bodywork specialists, massage therapists, cranio-sacral therapists, acupuncturists and Rolfers. Courses in Kiso Method™ are offered at the Traditional Chinese Medical College of Hawaii, the Kiso Life Healing Center in Hilo, Hawaii, through seminars, and online at www.KisoMethod.com; with international certification by Dr. Cain.

The **Kiso Method™** two-part manual is available in English or Japanese, translated by Hideko Russell, head professor of medical translation at the Monterey Institute of International Studies.

Dr. Cain has summarized the techniques of Kiso Method™ into a book designed for the lay-person, entitled **Secrets of Healing Back Pain**. This book is designed to enable an individual without medical *training to understand the causes of back pain, and more importantly, how to heal their own back pain. Exercises and stretches are shown, as well as use of the Kiso Ball, a device that helps a person manipulate their own back to rid the body of subluxation (bone out of place). **Secrets of Healing Back Pain** has also been translated into Japanese by Mrs. Russell.*

Dr. Cain has conducted seminars for over 20 years on health, wellbeing, healing back pain, and the Kiso Method™. Topics will now expand to include nutrition, weight loss and The Kiso Diet™.

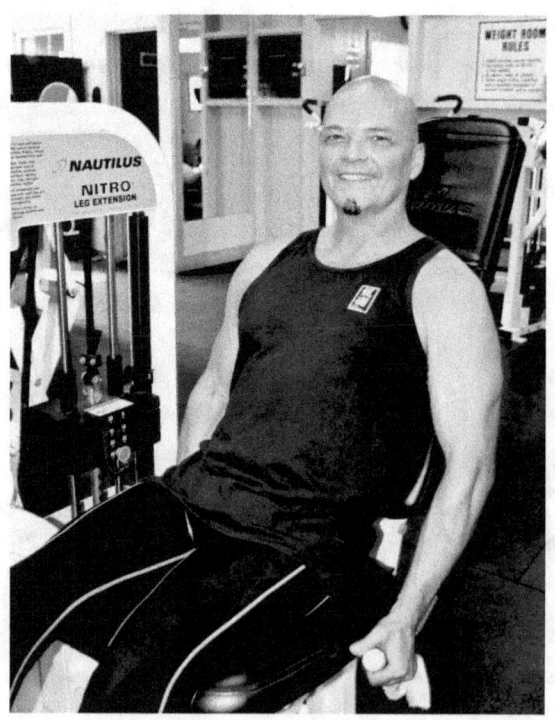